The Thinking Doctor

Observations on a Lifetime of Medicine

Ernest G. Warner, M.D.

THE ROADRUNNER PRESS
OKLAHOMA CITY, OKLAHOMA

For group sales, please contact
The RoadRunner Press at orders@theroadrunnerpress.com.

First edition December 2023
Printed in the United States of America.

Library of Congress Control Number: 2023951361

Names:
Warner, Ernest G., author.
Title:
The thinking doctor : observations on a wonderful lifetime of medicine /
Ernest G. Warner, M.D.
Description:
First edition. | Oklahoma City, Oklahoma : The RoadRunner Press, 2023.
Identifiers:
ISBN: 978-1-950871-26-1 (hardcover) | 978-1-950871-11-7 (trade paper) |
978-1-950871-27-8 (ePub) | 978-1-950871-28-5 (MOBI) | LCCN: 2023951361
Subjects:
LCSH: Warner, Ernest G. | Physicians--United States--Biography. | Med-
icine--United States. | Medical education--United States. | Physician and
patient. | BISAC: MEDICAL / History. | MEDICAL / Physicians. | MEDICAL /
Education & Training. | MEDICAL / Physician & Patient. | MEDICAL / Ethics.
Classification:
LCC: R154.W37 A3 2023 | DDC: 610.92--dc23

10 9 8 7 6 5 4 3 2 1

To my wife

*"The chapter you are learning today
is going to save someone's life tomorrow.
Pay attention."*
—Unknown

Preface

You will note as you begin this book that the first anecdote is not directly related to medicine. This is to demonstrate that before one becomes a compleat physician, one first needs to become a reasonably compleat mature man or woman. Knowledge of American society, how it acts, and how individuals interact in this world of increasing complexity is essential.

The purpose of this book is to relate for posterity the methodology for training physicians from roughly 1950 to recent years when computerization began to take over much of the functions of the teacher.

Personally, I find this a problem from the standpoint of teaching clinical medicine. I am a firm believer in the Socratic method of teaching in which the teacher, through questions and dialogue, engages with the student on a direct personal basis.

It is my hope that you will enjoy this book and come to understand how marked the transition of medicine has been from when I entered the profession to the modern electronic age we know now. As technology infringes on the student-teacher relationship, we risk losing the personal touch that has served medical students and our profession so well. Medicine can only ever be taught by study of the humanities and living out in the world—by this, I mean the nonmedical world where most of our patients exist on a daily basis. Why? Because if my years as a physician have taught me anything, it is that it is essential to understand the person and how that person's disease interacts with the patient individually.

This book is dedicated to my wife who has demonstrated great patience throughout my sixty-five years of neurological practice. She is the one who encouraged me repeatedly when I was ready to give up, chiding me with this simple reminder: "I married a doctor!"

My thanks also goes to my transcriptionist, Ellie Burns, who has tolerated my erratic style of dictating with great patience, and my daughter Susan Warner Reed Karther who saw this book to completion.

Ad majorem Dei gloriam.

Introduction

The purpose of this book is to chronicle how medicine was taught, learned, and practiced from 1951 to 2016. This was the time that I was in medical school, internship, residency, and private practice—as well as a spell in the military. Neurology has been my specialty.

This informal history is told in a series of anecdotes, which I share roughly in chronological order. Each story is individual but also illustrates both the experience and the adventure that medicine was in those days just past. Hopefully, these experiences can also serve as an historical record of sorts, and more importantly, go on to inspire a new generation of young physicians who have nothing but the most modern technology at their fingertips—none of which was known to us not too long ago.

When I say take yourself back to the early days of medicine, *early days* is not a misnomer. Medical history can be traced back to the Ancient Greeks, and one can learn a good bit about physicians, their caring, and their scientific investigations by studying the works of early doctors such as Louis Pasteur, Ignaz Semmelweis, Robert Koch, William Halstead, and William Osler.

As our story starts, take a moment to consider what was employed on a daily basis as I entered the American medical system:

1) There was no imaging—no magnetic resonance imaging or MRIs, CT or CAT scans, or ultrasounds.

2) Pregnancy tests were done with guinea pigs.

3) Every summer, epidemics of polio, or poliomyelitis, required the use of large Drinker tank respirators, or iron lungs.

4) There was no renal dialysis.

5) There were few hepatic function tests for analyzing cells in the liver.

6) There was no endoscopy. Also, there were not yet colonoscopy or endoscopic exams done as there were no flexible scopes! The technology simply didn't exist.

7) Cystoscopy was done with outside tubing of the cystoscope measuring about the size of an index finger. When inserted in the penis, the pain produced was severe, as this distorted the penile urethra.

8) The resectoscope to resect the prostate gland was even larger. (Think of that, gentlemen!)

9) There were no antibiotics save for penicillin. Only later would streptomycin come out, then chloromycetin, which is thought to have killed a good number of patients. Sulfa drugs came later.

10) There were no birth-control pills, intrauterine devices, or IUDs. No implanted contraceptives or intravaginal diaphragms. The only contraceptive available was abstinence—the simple

statement of the word, *No*—followed by the honoring of said statement.

11) Blood transfusions were given through rubber tubing, tubing that then went on to be used again and again for transfusions and with patients. The inability to adequately clean the tubes produced fever and chills in almost every patient. There was no disposable plastic tubing at the time. All injections were given using glass syringes. These were sterilized in an autoclave, and the needles were similarly re-sterilized by boiling. Urinary catheters were also re-sterilized.

12) There were no cardiac pacemakers or defibrillators, and electrocardiograms, or EKGs, were charted on paper—one piece of paper at a time.

13) There were *no transplants*—not renal, not cardiac, not lung. Such procedures had yet to be developed, and even if they had, no immunosuppressants were available to

remedy rejection of a transplanted organ.

14) The only cardiac medications available were morphine, mercurial diuretics, aminophylline, and digitalis. All modern medicines—particularly antihypertensives—were not available. For hypertension, we had phenobarbital or rauwolfia. The newer drugs that revolutionized the treatment of hypertension were yet to be invented.

15) Diabetes was treated with insulin and diet, as there was no other treatment. Dosage was regulated by testing the urine sugar. A reagent tablet was dropped into a test tube with urine. Depending on the color that developed, the dose of insulin was administered. That was the best we had for ordering treatment. Certainly we had no such blood sugar tests as are available now, much less insulin pumps.

16) There were no electronic records. (I find electronic records to be a mixed blessing. That is, while they improve record keeping,

they're not oriented toward patient care
as physicians understand the term. They
are oriented toward having computers
diagnose rather than a physician analyzing
the problem using his at-the-ready,
in-house computer: *the brain.*

17) There were no technological advances
in the laboratories—that is, the fourteen
tests now included in most comprehensive
metabolic panels to measure the different
substances in your blood did not exist
together. Instead, each test had to be
drawn and run individually.
   The laboratory turnaround time was long
—sometimes one or two days—whereas
results are now obtained within hours.

18) No effective treatment existed for cancer
save for surgery and radiation. Now, with
newer drugs, often cancer patients can
live for many years post diagnosis.

19) Hospital transport was not a 9-1-1 call
away from an ambulance service but

provided by undertakers using hearses. As you may well imagine, funeral directors were not trained in first aid, and some patients arrived at the hospital having inadvertently been handled quite poorly. Now there are full-time ambulance services with well-trained emergency medical technicians capable of rendering emergency care and even triage.

20) Working conditions for interns and residents in teaching hospitals have significantly improved. (I am not at all sure, however, that the teaching capabilities themselves improved with the new changes.)

21) In my first year out of medical school, at the old age of twenty-six, I received the princely sum of $100 a month, including free laundry, free meals, and six additional free meals for, quote, *guests*. The extra meals were meant to take care of one's social life—or, in my case, my wife, as we desperately needed to crimp where we could so as not to fall into the red.

22) Three years later, as a thirty-one-year-old senior resident, I was pocketing $175 a month. We barely scraped by on the stipend by the time rent was paid on a two-room apartment. Fortunately, my wife was a schoolteacher. She taught school throughout my medical schooling and most of my residency—until her first pregnancy with delivery in June 1958, followed by the second with delivery in September 1959. The point being that the amount of money paid was called a stipend, not a salary, for a reason. Now, residents are paid a more-than-adequate living wage and do not have to moonlight to make enough money to eat. I have to say, though, that the experience gained in moonlighting was at times equal to that gained in the hospital. One had the oppor-tunity to apply his or her medical knowledge learned in a teaching situation on a practical level—without supervision.

23) The hours worked in those days were incredible, and one learned simply to do

without sleep while also trying to sustain
cognitive function at a normal level.
A normal workday was from 7:00 a.m. to
6:00 p.m. When one was *on call*, which
was every other night as an intern, one
worked thirty-five hours: from 7:00 a.m.
one day to 6:00 p.m. the next day. This
was almost a normal forty-hour work
week in less than two days! After such
a shift, I remember falling into bed
and sleeping for ten hours straight.

24) When I was a neurology resident, there
was no *on call*. That is: For a solid year,
save for a two-week vacation, my shift was
twenty-four hours a day, seven days a week.
This was made possible in part by a
tunnel that connected the hospital with the
nearby apartment complex where the
residents lived. In the middle of the
night, a resident could travel via the
tunnel (remember, this was Chicago) and
not only be safe but also protected from
the frequent inclement winter weather of
the Windy City.

25) New rules now limit residents' time on call with mixed results. No longer can residents follow the natural course of a disease from start to finish—by diagnosing patients, treating said patients, and then observing the natural course of the disease or ailment on the patient. Such observations were once stored as part of a physician's permanent memory to be recalled later as needed. After all, the whole name of the medical game is learning to *practice* medicine—once done under supervision but often without much sleep. Today, I am shocked to hear that residents in the middle of an operation must step away in some instances because they have put in their allowed time. This is done to make sure residents get enough rest so that they can function without being sleep deprived—much as we do with long-haul truckers or airline pilots. However, in a hospital, this new rule can also interrupt the flow of physical learning by residents—and ignores the fact that sometimes medicine must be practiced in less than optimal

situations. The point being that the paradigm of protecting physicians from adversity brought on by the very practice of medicine automatically *decreases* the time spent with patients, which is when one *learns* medicine. Unfortunately, it is just a fact that much of such learning often occurs at 2:00 a.m. or 3:00 a.m. and not during the regular office hours observed by the rest of the world.

We will cover a lot of ground in the pages that follow. However, in the end, this book is not meant to be an exhaustive history of medicine but rather to illustrate some of the changes that took place over these past sixty-five years. The anecdotes included here are my own but also typical for the epoch.

It is my sincere hope that you will enjoy reading them and be thankful for how far medicine has come.

—Ernest G. Warner, M.D.
Edmond, Oklahoma
2023

Chapter One

Lessons Learned in Early Life

A S A TEENAGER, I worked in the buildings and grounds department at Wheaton College in Illinois. I was assigned to the painting crew, and specifically to a gentleman by the name of Mr. Cannon. Mr. Cannon exemplified the best of the German immigrants of that time. I never knew his first name, yet he taught me a lifelong lesson, one that I believe is worth repeating.

We were refinishing floors by hand, a tedious process involving hours on one's hands and knees. After finishing a particular tough spot, I got up from the floor and announced, "Well, that's good enough."

Mr. Cannon immediately stopped what he was doing and rose to his feet. He stood as straight and tall as he could, a grand total of about five feet, three inches.

"Please stand up," he said, which I quickly did.

He looked at me and said, "What did you just say?"

"I said that was 'good enough.' "

He replied, "There is no 'good enough.' There is only right or wrong, correct or incorrect, finished or not finished."

With that, he sent me back to recheck the work that I had done and to correct any errors or oversights that remained. Only then was I allowed to declare the job finished. His was a lesson I never forgot.

Many years later, when my father was laid out in a funeral home in Wheaton, Illinois, I was taken into the back of the mortuary by the funeral director. There I recognized instantly not only my father but also Mr. Cannon. These two significant men in my life were lying in adjacent coffins before me. Mr. Cannon was gone, but the lesson he had taught me remained, and it has served me well throughout my years as a doctor.

* * * * *

My medical career began on an early Saturday morning in the spring of 1951. I remember the moment well as it would change my life—at least the next sixty-five years of it. The occasion was the arrival of an acceptance letter from the Dean's office, University of Illinois Medical School, Chicago, Illinois. At the time, I lived in the Chicago suburb of Wheaton, and I had applied for medical school in a very bad year—a bad year because so many other people had also applied.

The school was faced with a glut of post-war GI bill applicants, predominantly veterans, men serious about pursuing their educational opportunities. Hence, the rate of acceptance to medical schools in the United States that year was estimated to be one in every twelve applicants. Most people were applying to several medical schools. I had applied only to one: the University of Illinois, where my friends had attended, where my allegiance laid, and where tuition was the cheapest!

With the acceptance letter came a carefully constructed list of books to be purchased before entering the hallowed halls of learning. These included *Gray's Anatomy*, weighing in at about five pounds—plus two equally weighty tomes on biochemistry and physiology as well as an *Atlas of Anatomy*. Altogether, my book purchases would add up to approximately one hundred dollars in 1951 dollars, the equivalent of about a thousand dollars today. Of possibly more importance, the books represented a significant amount of weight to carry to school for a commuter student. I obtained a large satchel to haul the books to and from my residence to the medical school, laboratories, library, and places beyond. Thus began my lifetime journey in the practice of medicine, and what would later become a focus in neurology and electroencephalography.

Chapter Two

Anatomy

OF ALL THE COURSES of the freshman year for a medical student, anatomy must be simultaneously the most startling, impressive, and discouraging. You are faced with learning all the intricacies of structure and morphology of the human body, both male and female, along with the extremely variable arrangements of *anomalous* anatomy, or that which does not follow the textbook *normal* pattern. To say the least, it is intimidating. The idea of mastering the structure of bones, arteries, veins, lymphatic systems, and central and peripheral nervous systems seems an impossible task—much less doing so in only nine months.

The standard anatomy textbook, *Gray's Anatomy*, is about three inches thick and must be accompanied by the *Atlas of Dissections of the Human Body*. As one progresses in

the dissection of the cadaver, the findings are closely cor-
related with what one sees in the *Atlas* and also the more
academic, pedantic approach of *Gray's Anatomy*—thousands
of relationships to become familiar with—and that was just
for one freshman course.

The Anatomy Department provided each of us with a
bone box: a wooden latched box that contained one of each
of the major bones in the human body for our study at
home. Our bone boxes made for let's just say interesting
situations. Several of us commuted from the western suburbs of Chicago on the Aurora and Elgin Railroad, known
locally as the Great Third Rail until its abrupt closure of
passenger service in 1957. The train could take us to the
medical center in inner Chicago in about an hour.

One day as we were quietly riding and studying notes
(that is, memorizing various lists of names for nerves,
bones, insertions, origins of muscles and the like), an unfortunate event for one individual (delightful for the rest
of us) occurred: One of the boxes opened, and the bones
spilled out and into the aisle. What then ensued on the
crowded commuter train was horrifying—daily commut-
ers do not expect to see human bones rolling around on
the floor or down the aisle of their train car. Fortunately,
enough of us medical students were on hand that we quickly got the bones back in their box. Even more fortunate,

no one on the train decided to report our peer as a lunatic, a murderer, or someone worthy of police attention.

The actual anatomy laboratory was a cold, cavernous, gray-colored room that emanated death. Located on the top floor of the building, skylights dotted the ceiling, providing the best natural light supply one could procure. The view of Chicago from the anatomy laboratory was beautiful too, although you couldn't have told it by our behavior. We kept our focus mainly directed on what was happening inside the laboratory and with the remains of the dead bodies we were methodically disassembling.

Each cadaver was suspended on a platform inside a coffin-shaped metal box. The lid was bisected in the middle. When one opened both halves, the cadaver was raised to the surface, which then allowed one to conveniently and easily do dissections.

Cadavers were preserved with phenol or carbolic acid. The unfortunate effect of this preservative was that all of us reeked of phenol. Spouses were less than entranced with this odor, especially the ones who washed our laboratory coats. The phenol also rendered our fingertips rather anesthetic, which decreased the perception of what we were doing with them. The numbness wore off by the succeeding morning, and was only a minor handicap to the actual work involved. At the close of the anatomy session, the two halves of the cadaver container were closed, and, once again, order and some degree of decorum were restored.

Four freshman students were assigned to each cadaver. I was joined by a young woman of Asian descent, an older man (probably in his early thirties) who was married with several children, and a single gentleman named Ken. Ken and I were assigned to the left side of the body; the other two students, to the right. On occasion, our teams would assist each other across the body, but when we worked on the extremities, we would be reasonably independent.

Unfortunately, and rather tragically, within several weeks our two cadaver partners were no longer with us. As had been pointed out in the introductory session to medical school, approximately 20 percent to 30 percent of students would flunk out before the end of the freshman year. For that reason, every day one felt the sword dangling over one's neck wondering who might be next. A month had yet to pass, and Ken and I were now experiencing the reality of that statistic as we were left to do the dissection on the entire cadaver by ourselves.

Then Ken became quite ill with a severe case of infectious mononucleosis that was bad enough to require hospitalization. On the positive side, with the help of my notes and his assiduous studying, Ken managed to keep up with his studies and graduate with our class.

The Thinking Doctor

*****

A most interesting feature of the school's anatomy laboratory was the lab assistant whom I will call Wilhelm (not his actual name). Wilhelm was a man solely dedicated to the care of cadavers. This was his entire life from morning until night—24/7. Wilhelm was not very bright—and that was quite obvious to all. The story that followed him was that when he was a young boy, his father had brought him to the big city from their home in rural Illinois. Their destination: the Medical Center Anatomy Department. The exact connections that made what happened next possible are not known or lost to history, but Wilhelm was presented to the Professor of Anatomy, and this professor promised to give Wilhelm a job and take care of him. The professor did just that, as did subsequent heads of the department. One of those anatomy professors even made sure that Wilhelm had an occasional case of beer and otherwise looked after his physical well-being. Wilhelm never married, but the story had one last twist. Upon his death, the man from whom little had been expected but much had been given repaid the generosity of the University of Illinois by leaving an extremely large sum of money to the school in his will—a reminder of the folly in judging anyone by appearances.

*****

Since the first year of medical school was dedicated to the study of the anatomy and functions of the human body under normal conditions, part of the curriculum covered physiology as well as biochemistry. One of our physiology professors was a formidable six-foot, six-inch tall former German dirigible pilot who walked with his head tilted back and his eyes forever scanning the horizon. We assumed he was looking for enemy planes—a habit possibly leftover from his time in the zeppelin or dirigible service of the Luftwaffe, or German air force, of the Third Reich, or Wehrmacht. The man rarely interacted with students, which was fortunate since we represented his not so long ago enemies from World War II!

If the former German dirigible pilot turned medical school professor ignored us, the same could not be said for our German professor of neuroanatomy. We had fascinating interchanges with Dr. Heidrich von Himmel, a self-professed and propagandizing atheist. He accepted 110 percent of all claims regarding the theory of evolution—even the ones which gave some pause. With equal vigor, Himmel rejected any notion of metaphysics or God. In the course of one lecture, he declared there could not be any sort of *Almighty/God/Designer* given that all the intricate parts of the human body had evolved by evolution. This was a settled issue in his mind. Any student who took exception with this in any way, big or small, was deemed ignorant, unlearned, and probably unteachable by him. This was despite the fact that a number of us had a religious or at least a philosophical background in which other viewpoints were entertained or held.

Unfortunately, ours could not be proved by simple measurements of weight, length, height, or depth, and our professor's final sally was that the Bible said, God made Eve out of one of Adam's ribs, however if you count the ribs in males, you will find that they have a full set. (If the Biblical account is true, they should have only eleven.)

We thrived on the exchanges with our professor while remaining puzzled at the theories of a man with a mindset formed in prejudice rather than reason. That is, the genetics of a person remain intact despite losing one rib or one leg. In other words, when that individual breeds with another, the genetic makeup produces a completely normal individual, with twelve ribs for both males and females. This seemed an obvious flaw to our professor's theory. Of course, one could not raise it with this particular professor as he was much too erudite and quick to deflect. His obvious disdain for those below him in the pecking order (and we were as low as one could get) didn't help.

*****

One of the most influential figures for us at the time was a senior lecturer in gross anatomy, a Dr. Zimmerman. Dr. Zimmerman had an encyclopedic knowledge of the human anatomy, and his lectures were displays of overt creative genius. He was known to present the material on an old-fashioned blackboard using a range of colors of chalk. Red was used for arteries. Blue, for veins, with nerves in green, and bone in yet another color. He was ambidextrous, so he would simultaneously draw anatomic structures with red chalk in one hand and blue chalk in the other.

We would be drawing furiously with ink pen or pencil as he presented the structures and their relationship through the human body—say a nerve that went over an artery, or between an artery and a vein, or under a vein—such behavior had to be learned as a matter of dictum.

There were not several but thousands of such body parts to be carefully cataloged and memorized, including not only structures like the muscles but also all the various names, most of which were in Latin. This became an interesting example of learning on the job and struggling in the process. Each night we would decipher our notes using the *Atlas of Anatomy* and *Gray's Anatomy* in an attempt to make sense out of the day's lecture and blackboard drawings. We then memorized it so as to be able to retrieve and regurgitate the information on the test that we knew with certainty would come at the end of the semester. I have never seen another person who could sketch human anatomy like Dr. Zimmerman. Fortunately, he had a habit of leaving his masterpieces on the board each day so that we had the opportunity to copy them later.

One of the more interesting perks of the anatomy course was having access to the Anatomy Department Museum. This held preserved specimens on display for those who needed to study such material. Multiple large jars (about the size of a five-gallon bucket) held the whole bodies of infant corpses with severe congenital anomalies. Most of us mentioned these exhibits to our wives/girlfriends/fiancées. We never gave it a second thought; it was just part of our learning experience.

What did surprise us, however, was when most of our girlfriends then said that they wanted to *see* these pregnancies that had gone wrong. I have never been able to understand why a woman who is pregnant would want to be exposed to the sight of helpless malformed infants that did not make it. Nonetheless, the women I have known seemed to have a morbid curiosity to see what might happen in the course of a pregnancy! Oh, the intricacies of the female mind that have never been explained and probably never will be. (Perhaps males are better off not understanding how female minds work. Pardon the philosophical comments, but in medicine one necessarily develops a good number of philosophical concepts after observing the breadth of human behavior.)

Chapter Three

Pharmacology

PHARMACOLOGY WAS TAUGHT in the second year of medical school. These drug demonstrations embedded themselves in our minds, possibly because along with the written and spoken materials we saw the effects of the medications on live animals.

There were a good number of anti-vivisectionists in the community at the time, and they would occasionally burst into the laboratory in the middle of an experiment in an attempt to rescue the animals being operated on. It was difficult to convince these folks that it was better to experiment on animals than on human beings. They seemed quite inured to the concept of science being scientific and based on experimental activities. All of the animals that were used were from various dog pounds or supply houses. The animals were carefully anesthetized so that they suffered no pain during the experiment. The experiments did usually terminate their lives, but animals that would have been put to death in a dog pound otherwise, would have done so with no benefit to humankind.

Ethically speaking, this is utilitarian reasoning. It is also reasoning that must be used with great care or it can become an excuse for unethical behavior. The doctors in Nazi Germany demonstrated this with their embrace of eugenics during the Holocaust.

Chapter Four

Cook County Hospital

DURING ONE OF MY medical clerkships during the last two years of medical school in Illinois, I was delighted to have a rotation at what was then the Cook County Hospital. The place housed thousands of patients at any given time, and the hospital even had one floor where chronic neurological patients lived out their lives.

The trade-off of the arrangement was obvious: In exchange for a home and full medical maintenance, the patients lived together as a teaching example for medical students. Keeping them in this museum-like situation was helpful to them from both a research and treatment standpoint. In those days, this was also considered a fair trade-off for society as the diseases that the patients had were often congenital or rare conditions. I am sure now such institutional warehousing would likely be deemed barbaric. Yet one should be slow to judge what occurred decades before in a different time and under different societal circumstances.

*****

Like most work places, Cook County Hospital had its feuds. One of the ongoing ones was between Dr. Roker and Dr. Dean, two equally brilliant professors. Dr. Rocker was a respected internist; Dr. Dean, a senior professor in the Pathology Department. The two men held clinical pathological conferences every week or two, and we attended them as part of our medical education.

The professors were a delight to watch, especially when they commenced verbally fencing with each other. The pathologist's edge was he got to examine the dead body, so his would be the final word when it came to any diagnosis. The internist's job was to use the patient's full clinical record prior to death to ascertain the correct diagnosis *before* the autopsy. I never saw Dr. Roker make a single mistake or miss a single diagnosis. This was known to infuriate Dr. Dean because quite often Dr. Roker was known to find unusual and rare cases, such as rare tropical diseases (in Chicago!) or strange allergic reactions.

The demography of Cook County Hospital was also fascinating in its own right as it is in all hospitals. At the time, infectious diseases were still very extant, and medical students often acted as part-time nurses. I worked as a nurse in the hospital's infectious disease building two evenings a week. This gave me an opportunity to observe a number of infectious diseases that would not otherwise have crossed my path. A great source of pride for me has always been that I have actually seen *several* cases of diphtheria. There are only rare physicians in the United States living now who have seen even a single case.

The infectious disease unit saw multiple cases of meningitis of all types, including pneumococcus, meningococcal, and other infectious agents (now rare cases) of chickenpox (varicella); generalized herpes zoster virus; and multiple cases of scarlet fever, whooping cough (pertussis), smallpox (variola), and measles.

There were also yearly outbreaks of poliomyelitis, or polio, the dread disease of children in particular that produced crippling paralysis. As you may recall, President Franklin Delano Roosevelt was a victim of the polio virus. Despite intensive physical therapy, he needed leg braces to walk. He was never heard to complain about this, at least not publicly. Some of the wards in which I worked in those days were filled with cases of poliomyelitis.

One night I reported for duty at 11:00 p.m. only to walk into a ward containing six patients on respirators. In those days, the only way for patients paralyzed by polio to breathe was to put them in a Drinker mechanical respirator (popularly known as an iron lung) that breathed for them. These large green metal tanks had ports on the sides through which one would insert arms to facilitate nursing care, including providing a bed pan or giving medication shots. Being in a respirator and unable to move could produce bedsores, or decubitus ulcers, unless the patients were turned frequently.

Other frequent complications for polio patients included pneumonia and electrolyte imbalances. If they could not swallow, having bulbar poliomyelitis, they would have feeding tubes inserted to provide liquid nourishment and other fluids. Most patients did not get bulbar polio but rather had problems with paralysis of their extremities (polio particularly affected lower levels of the spinal cord). If they had bulbar polio affecting the brain stem, the respiratory center would be affected. There was also frequent paralysis of the chest wall and diaphragm. The way the Drinker machine operated was by way of bellows that forced air in and out of the tank. When air entered the closed chamber, the chest would partially collapse, mimicing exhalation, and when the bellows produced negative pressure, the chest would inflate, mimicking normal inspiration. With six respirators and only one nurse to operate them, if the electricity stopped for any reason, a choice had to be made as to which individual to save. This was because the bellows had to be hand-pumped by a nurse. (I always made the choice at the beginning of my shift, after ascertaining which patient was most likely to survive in such a situation.)

One had to make a choice.

I emphasize this because many laypeople do not realize physicians sometimes are called to make such hard choices—choices between patients, some of whom will not survive because of those choices.

At Cook County, we once faced an entire ward of cases of pertussis (whooping cough). The eight-hour routine ran from 11:00 p.m. to 7:00 a.m. It started at one end of the room with eight to ten babies: changing diapers, giving antibiotics, and making sure all of the babies had fluids running subcutaneously or intravenously. One would listen for the distinctive sound of whooping respiration, a sound which once heard one never forgets and one which I do hope that the reader will never hear.

Thankfully, pertussis can be prevented with immunization. However, with some parents becoming adverse to vaccines or neglectful when it comes to keeping their child's vaccinations up to date, this might not always be the case in the U.S.

Unless one has had reason to care for a baby with whooping cough, he or she might not realize how violent the cough associated with this respiratory illness is compared to a run-of-the-mill cough from the flu. With whooping cough, as the baby starts to hack, the force of the exertion can push both urine and feces out, necessitating frequent diaper changes. Some children may not cough at all but rather struggle to breath—or temporarily stop breathing. Whooping cough can also cause extreme fatigue in a child; a contagious bacterial disease chiefly affecting children, it is not something to take lightly.

In my early career, I also witnessed and treated cases of diphtheria, so I knew the threat that it could pose. One case was in a child; one, in an adult. The adult was a physician who had performed the autopsy on a child who had died of diphtheria. In the process, he became inoculated with diphtheria bacillus and developed an overt case. I was the only resident in internal medicine who noticed the false membrane that had formed in his throat. When I attempted to scrape it, he quickly declared, "I don't want anybody to look at my throat except the attending doctor!" (If I had been in his place, I would have said the same thing.) Fortunately, he lived.

Diphtheria is a preventable disease in the U.S., but we may again see diphtheria on the rise if people fail to take the need for immunization seriously.

One of the more interesting clinical professors during my training was a Dr. Moley, the master diagnostician at Cook County Hospital. Dr. Moley was a fascinating individual on a personal as well as a scientific level; he was also an excellent teacher. That said, he seemed oblivious to many social niceties. He dressed like an indigent. His shirts were usually tattered at the collars and cuffs. His ties were rumpled, if not dirty, and carelessly tied. His suit coat looked as if he had slept in it for at least a week as did his slacks, and his shoes were unpolished and scuffed. He was known to speak distinctly and slowly (some would say ploddingly) when explaining clinical problems, and in all the time we spent listening to him, we *never* witnessed him make a single mistake or become overtly excited.

One of Dr. Moley's more unusual clinical practices was how he performed rectal examinations. While we all made a point to always wear gloves and make sure said gloves had no holes, he did rectal examinations with his bare fingers. When asked why, Dr. Moley had a pragmatic response, "Because you can feel the anatomy much better than through a glove." He, of course, was again correct but I would posit there are other things to consider.

From a teaching standpoint, my experiences at Cook County Hospital were all a future doctor could want, and two of my cases there remain among the most interesting of my career.

The first involved a man approximately sixty years old who apparently had been drinking and fallen asleep. His bed caught on fire, and he was severely burned—on his legs, particularly. Somehow he did not succumb in the fire. He made it to the hospital where he was treated, and then transferred to the surgical ward where we took over his care. The intern to whom I was assigned had me help the patient each day by changing the dressings on his wounds. The old dressings came off saturated with thick, green, extremely malodorous pus—otherwise referred to as purulent exudate. We would then wash the wounds and redress them. Despite our best efforts, however, he eventually died. Skin grafting was in its infancy in those days, and he was unable to fight off a severe infection.

The other case may well offend some readers, but it is a case I will never forget. This gentleman came in with advanced stage penile cancer—that is, cancer of the penis. The odor produced by the cancer was sickening, and the sight of what it had done to the patient's body mirrored the smell. The man had open ulcerated wounds across both groins exuding abundant bloody exudate. His penis looked like a piece of cauliflower, and it was then that I realized why: he was uncircumcised.

Despite penile cancer being rare in North America—diagnosed in fewer than one man in a hundred thousand each year, most doctors are insistent when it comes to recommending circumcision. Seeing one case of advanced penile cancer, I am sure, would convince most parents too.

It surely did me.

Chapter Five

Physiology

IN 1951, DOCTORS HAD no oscilloscopes to analyze electronic signals in the body, no heart-lung machines for cardiopulmonary bypass, and no computers—basically none of the modern technology now available to physicians. Hence, the methodology in use to record physiological data in 1951 consisted of a smoked drum.

A smoked drum was a large loop of paper—approximately a foot and a half wide and eight feet long—that was carefully rotated by hand over a smoking lamp, which produced a layer of black soot that was placed on drums and a roller. The data being measured was input with a stylus, and the oscillations of the stylus was scratched onto the sooted surface. The drum rotated quite rapidly, so it was a means of recording rapidly changing physiological data.

At the close of the experiment, which was limited by the length of the drum and the speed with which it rotated, the drum was dipped into a bath of diluted shellac and dried. This preserved the record in a fashion that could then be handled. Measurements were taken and a comparison made between that experiment and others with different parameters—to say it was a primitive method would be to understate the basic technology behind it.

However rudimentary, the technology *did* work, which compensated somewhat for the fact that those of us who used it were left looking like soot-dusted chimney sweeps in formerly white coats.

Modern technology has since rendered this archaic.

Chapter Six

Pathology

MY GROSS PATHOLOGY course in our sophomore year started with my first autopsy. The procedure was done in a cold, damp amphitheater built with steeply pitched rows of seats to ensure a good view of the dissection taking place below. I arrived early. A large man, recently deceased, laid on the glistening stainless steel autopsy table. The dark, cavernous room was silent save for the distant sounds of traffic. On the wall above this rather dismal scene, in Latin, were the words:

Here the living learn from the dead.

It seemed a fitting start for my first pathology experience, which on this day would involve learning from the dead with systematic, studied dissection, removal, and examination of the deceased's internal organs.

The prosector, or pathology professor, appeared, reached for a scalpel, and deftly started to slice open the abdomen of the corpse. He lectured as he cut. He then reached for the rib cutters, which resembled loppers used for pruning trees. Each rib was individually cut, and with each cut came an echoing *crunch*. The anterior rib cage was then reflected upward, giving exposure to the heart and lungs.

As the professor dissected and then removed the various organs, each was weighed and taken elsewhere for further study. The tissues would be fixed, or pickled, and sliced into thin slices with a microtome. These would be stained according to the type of pathology suspected and used to demonstrate the microscopic anatomy. This made the gross pathology available and understandable on a microscopic basis.

Pathology is the basis of all medicine.

The abnormal structure of organs altered by disease is the *sine qua non* of understanding the effect of illness on the human body. Our job was to take the history, physical examination, and autopsy findings and put them into a formal case report (one report from each of us for academic credit) explaining how the pathology caused the observed pathophysiology changes in, for instance, blood constituents or changes on X-ray. This rendered a complete picture of the individual disease, or diseases, that had killed the patient. Our grade rested on the accuracy and relevance of the report. I found each case a worthy and interesting challenge.

This was truly the living learning from the dead, and I was one of the still living and learning.

Chapter Seven

Sophomore Year

DURING MY SOPHOMORE year, my bachelor Uncle Lada became quite ill. I went to visit him along with my family. My uncle had been a chronic alcoholic, but had recently quit the drink, so the heavy ingestion of ethyl alcohol had ceased. Nonetheless, he now had become quite ill with a fever and cough. The family physician, who had known my uncle as a drunk all these many years, declared the new illness another outcome of Uncle Lada's heavy drinking—he could not do anything for him.

Being a curious young medical student, I found myself perplexed by my uncle's symptoms, which did not seem to fit those of alcoholic complications. He had a fever and cough, which sounded more like either a cardiac or pulmonary problem to me. Now remember, I was only a sophomore medical student, not much more experienced than the average person on the street. Nonetheless, I put a stethoscope to Uncle Lada's chest and immediately recognized the sound of a large number of rales, a peculiar crackling that sounds like Rice Krispies crunching and popping. Rales usually signify inflammation or fluid in the lungs. I had some antibiotics available (not necessarily the correct ones), and put him on what I had, thinking I could certainly get in trouble if I were observed doing so. Sadly, before the antibiotics could have any effect, he died.

The next day I went to class and told one of the senior pathology professors, a member of the coroner's staff of the county, about his case. I pointed out that I did not believe he died of alcoholic complications. The professor responded, "Well, do you want to do an autopsy on him?"

"Well . . . I think that would be reasonable."

He said, "I do too. Where is the funeral home?"

I told him the location, and he said, "I will meet you there at 2:00 this afternoon."

I arrived at the appointed time at the funeral home and went into the mortuary where the embalmed body of my uncle was on the embalmer's table. The professor arrived with the necessary instruments and handed a scalpel to me. I gulped several times, having assumed that he would be the one doing the autopsy.

"No, you are going to do the autopsy," he said.

"Okay," I replied.

With that, I took the scalpel and slit my uncle's abdomen down the midline. There was no blood or body movement, but this gave us exposure to the abdominal cavity. I made two long incisions to the rib cage, then used a pair of long-handled nippers to cut open the rib cage. Ribs were cut individually on both sides, and after dissecting the soft tissue away, the plate of the ribs and breast bone (or sternum) were reflected upward en masse. We now had access to the chest with good visualization.

We removed the heart next and carefully scrutinized the organ. There was no evidence of any sort of major scar or other lesion present on the heart. The heart was anatomically normal for his age, with only some slight atherosclerosis, or hardening, present in the arteries. We then came to the lungs, and there we found the cause of his death. We had had some warning, because as we cut the lungs, a dense area in one lung could be felt. When we cut into the area, it exuded purulent fluid, or pus.

"Well that is what killed him," the professor said. "He had pneumonia."

Now remember that pneumonia in those days, while treatable, could often be fatal. Armed with a diagnosis, we put the body back together. I thanked the professor, and we bid each other adieu. I am sure the professor thought this experience would turn me into a pathologist, and that is why he so freely offered his services!

As for my uncle, I now had information that proved he had died of pneumonia and not liver disease. What was I to do with it? Store it away in memory?

Would it have done any good to approach that trusted WWII-decorated family physician about his error in judgment over the telephone? I didn't think so then, and I don't think so now. After all, it was after the fact. There are just some things that you, as a physician, have to evaluate and live with the rest of your life.

Chapter Eight

Psychiatry

IN OUR THIRD YEAR of medical school, we began to learn by doing and being involved in clinical situations in the hospital. We took histories and did physicals on the patients with the goal of making a diagnosis. That diagnosis would then be explored with the attending physician and possibly the house staff. Through this process we were taught but also challenged and corrected in our thinking.

Our psychiatry class consisted of twelve students. We each examined different patients with the help of a psychiatrist who knew all of their histories intimately. The psychiatrist was a female, full professor, and the author of the textbook we used in the course. After visiting with our patients, we would gather around a conference table with Dr. Mosselman at the head. The psychiatry professor asked us one by one what we had observed and how we would correlate that with the patient and diagnosis under discussion.

During one such session, I happened to be the last one in the rotation and maybe a too honest observer. I told the professor that—in my opinion—the patient's asthma was due to the entrance of male pollen, or sperm, into her bronchial tree, which the patient's system had then rejected. This had psychologically caused a bronchospasm, producing a clinical case of asthma. My diagnosis was psychoanalysis straight out of Dr. Masselman's own textbook!

The professor's response was to ask me where I had gone to school—a rather perplexing and irrelevant question it seemed to me. Nonetheless, I told her that I had gone to Wheaton College, in Wheaton, Illinois, a conservative Christian liberal arts college. At this, she declared, "Oh, you are in deep trouble. . . . I will counsel with you and help you get through this!"

As far as I was concerned, my only psychological problem was being chronically sleep-deprived from working the night shift. Dr. Masselman would not relent and demanded that I remain after class for a one-on-one consult. I politely declined, explaining that my only concerns in life were staying awake and getting enough money to finish medical school. This did not go over well.

Remember, Dr. Masselman was a full professor of psychiatry and the author of the textbook that we were using—a textbook from which I had gotten the information for my diagnosis. I do not remember what grade she gave me in that class, but I never heard another word about my need for counseling or psychiatric help.

*****

One of the most interesting areas of psychiatry to me was the use of electric shock treatment. While there are pros and cons of such treatment, when it comes to some forms of severe depression (it was called involutional melancholia in those days), electric shock can be extremely effective. The downside, however, is that occasionally during the convulsion, unmodified electric shock treatment (EST) can also break bones.

When administering the procedure, the electrodes were placed on both sides of the patient's skull, and then electricity was passed between the electrodes to produce a tonic-clonic, or severe, convulsion. During the convulsion, the movements of the limbs were severe, resulting in occasional breaks, particularly in the arms and sometimes in the legs. For obvious reasons, fractured bones secondary to treatment for profound depression is undesirable for both the patient and the physician. (It has, however, made some malpractice lawyers rich.)

Having already been trained in anesthesia, one day I asked Dr. Avery, "Why don't you try giving some muscle relaxants to these people before you give them the shock? If we paralyze them, at least they won't be breaking bones!"

He looked at me rather quizzically, thought about it for a few moments, and said, "Can you do that, Warner?"

Being more sure of myself than I should have been, I replied, "Oh, of course" or something to that effect.

"Good! We will do it tomorrow morning!"

I was already regretting opening my mouth.

Nonetheless, the next morning we tried out my theory on our very first patient, a fairly robust man (that is, one with good muscle development) who might be likely to break bones during a hard convulsion.

We gave the patient enough sodium pentothal to produce a mild degree of unconsciousness without depressing his respiration. We then also gave him a dose of succinylcholine, which depolarized his muscles and produced a flaccid patient, unable to move. We immediately put an oxygen mask on his face and inflated his lungs repeatedly with the tank of oxygen, so he was well oxygenated and looked pink. In those days there were no oximeters to measure blood oxygen saturation or any other kind of monitors for this situation. The only monitor we had was our fingers on his pulse and a stethoscope on his heart. We had electrocardiogram leads on his chest, and as soon as the convulsions stopped, we would hook him up to the machine so that we could get a single strip of EKG.

For those of you wondering, it was a single lead of EKG, not the twelve-or-more-lead EKGs that are now obtained simultaneously.

With these primitive measures to protect the patient's oxygen supply and his brain, we proceeded to shock him. The result was a few tiny muscle twitches in his feet and no overt convulsion. When the twitching stopped, we inflated his lungs again with oxygen and watched his EKG, monitoring all of his vital signs. After the usual period of post-electric shock stupor, the patient woke up improved.

After that, Dr. Avery wanted all of his patients treated in this manner. In retrospect, we used the best technique possible at the time based on our understanding of the physiology of what we were doing. Nowadays, this would be considered overt malpractice given the lack of adequate monitoring and safeguards. In those days, however, there was nothing else to do. Without electric shock treatment, many of the patients would have become increasingly depressed and nonfunctional. I should hasten to add that electric shock treatment is now always done with this type of protection against overt seizures—but with much better agents, better monitoring, and better technique. To my knowledge, we were the first to try it at the time, and we did so in one of the major hospitals in Chicago.

*****

One of the differences in medicine in the earlier years was that Neurology and Psychiatry were combined. That is, I was a neurology resident and I also ran a closed and locked psychiatry ward where I was involved in the care of a large number of patients—many of them either violent or psychotic.

I never felt threatened by any of these patients though, nor was I ever assaulted by any of them. I could walk into a room where a person was screaming threats and swinging at the nurses, sit down on the patient's bed, and start up a conversation. Almost without exception (for reasons that still elude me), the patients would give me a rather startled look and then start to talk, or at least to listen.

Several of them would go on to give me intricately made hot-plate holders as presents, presents that I still have to this day. I have never been sure why I had such a good rapport with these patients. Perhaps because I was a little crazy myself? Or perhaps because they somehow knew they could safely confide in me? I suspect the latter, and that it had something to do with my never being in a rush and always being willing to take the time to listen to them. I do, however, remember one exception to this.

Dr. Marvin, a neurologist and my immediate chief, was in a room waiting for a patient. The room was narrow and the patient entered from one end. We were sitting at the opposite end of this closed room with Dr. Marvin in a chair, smoking his perpetual cigarette, and me sitting on a cot. The patient no more came in than he began to scream and holler threats. Naked from the waist up, he had the muscle development of the American bodybuilder Charles Atlas. In other words, he could have leveled either one of us with one or two blows, but it was obvious to everyone that he was headed for Dr. Marvin.

Dr. Marvin was a calm, thin, laconic person. As the patient approached him, Dr. Marvin sat quietly, with his knees crossed and a cigarette between his fingers. As the patient descended on him, the good doctor took a drag on his cigarette and exhaled, forcefully blowing smoke in the patient's face. The patient wilted, collapsing on the other end of the cot from me.

Dr. Marvin never uttered a word to the patient. He simply picked up where he had left off in his conversation with me. The event might as well have never happened.

To this day, I do not understand how Dr. Marvin knew that blowing smoke in the patient's face would stop the man in his tracks. Today this would, at the very least, be considered bad manners.

Chapter Nine

Obstetrics, Gynecology, Prenatal-Infant Loss

OBSTETRICS AND GYNECOLOGY when I was a medical student were divided into third- and fourth-year medical clerkships. Third-years practiced at Cook County Hospital, which, on average, saw a thousand babies delivered a month—primarily of working poor and indigent patients who could not afford private care. Fourth-years practiced at a suburban hospital outside Chicago that was strictly filled with upper-class private patients.

At Cook County, we worked twelve-hour shifts with a team of ob/gyn residents in training. Being junior medical students, we were the low rung. Our main job was to prevent a precipitous delivery, or the abrupt delivery of babies in the bed as opposed to on the delivery table where it was safer if an emergency developed.

Unfortunately, no matter how careful we were, every one of us had at least one case that led to precipitous delivery, despite routine cervical checks. The cervix, or mouth of the uterus that widens during labor, has to dilate enough to get as much of the infant's head through as possible before the actual delivery. Our job was to check every hour to be sure that at the moment in which the cervix was thinned, widened, and delivery was imminent, the patient was whisked into the delivery suite.

The predelivery area was divided into two parts: The first had six beds and was for *primips*, a woman having her first baby. There was absolutely no privacy for the patients, as both this ward and the ward for *multips*, a woman who had previously delivered a child, had no walls or even curtains. While this may seem barbaric, it provided safety and good observation of each individual patient in labor. If a patient took a turn, the change would be recognized immediately and emergency procedures instituted—for both the mother and the infant if need be.

During this twelve-hour shift, we did histories and physical examinations of the patients. We were rushed beyond belief; our shifts followed by collapse and then twelve hours off. This hospital's delivery rate of one thousand infants a month averaged out to about thirty a day, or more than one per hour.

As might be expected, multiple complications arose, as most of the patients had received no prenatal care; the benefit of the delivery area setup became clear at such times. If a patient required an emergency Cesarean section, the procedure could be done in a space immediately adjacent to the delivery table, where a full surgical setup was instantly available.

The second week, we spent time on the delivery line with most of us actually delivering babies. It fell to us to deliver all of the *multips*, while the delivery of the first-time mothers was left to the experienced residents. This made good sense. (Once a vaginal delivery occurs through the birth canal without incident, it's generally accepted that another could take place without a problem.)

That wasn't always the case. One day I successfully delivered a baby, resuscitated it, clamped the cord, and then looked back at the mother only to still see a large mass in her lower abdomen. Clearly, another baby was present. I informed the patient and screamed for the resident on duty, who came immediately. The resident moved the patient to an area where more equipment was available, and delivered the second baby. This was a memorable example of the lack of adequate prenatal medical care being given to these indigent women, as the mother had no idea she was carrying twins.

The next morning, the job of the medical students was to make the rounds of all the women who had delivered the previous day and draw blood samples from them. Specifically, we were checking them for anemia and syphilis, but the screening also took place for other diseases that might be present. HIV was unknown in those days.

I will never forget the visual of twenty patients spread across a big room waiting with their arms out to have blood drawn. Most of the patients were black, and finding veins in black skin can be somewhat of a challenge at first. However, by the end of a week of this routine, one becomes quite adept at finding even small or reluctant veins and extracting adequate blood from them. As a third-year medical student and prospective future doctor, you would have been considered a failure if by then you failed to find a vein in each and every woman in the ward.

Our second ob/gyn rotation was at a private hospital in the suburbs of Chicago. Our main jobs there were to observe, assist, and do histories; physical examinations; and evaluation of laboratory work. At this point in medical school, we were considered an essential part of the medical team, and our opinions were taken into consideration in the forming of most medical judgments.

Two instances come to mind in which I was involved in a personal way. The first occurred at approximately

2:00 a.m. on what had started as a quiet shift at the hospital until a patient began screaming in distress. She was about to deliver.

The attending physician was a much older general practitioner who rarely did deliveries. I was assisting him. Unfortunately, it became obvious that this patient had not received an adequate episiotomy—a local incision to widen the birth canal and prevent tearing—and so had deeply torn her vaginal wall. At 0200 there was the GP, me, and two nurses manning the unit. The GP could not stop the blood flow from the tear, and I could see quite clearly that the patient was going to exsanguinate, or be drained of blood, if we did not take fast action.

I told the nurse to start fluids at a high rate of flow to try to maintain blood pressure, and then asked for a curved needle and a needle holder with sutures. The GP looked at the mess in front of us and asked if I could "do anything." I luckily had a fair idea, having taken part in many deliveries by this point.

I took the needle holder and started at the apex of the tear, closed the wound there, and then did the same thing lower in the wound with a running stitch. The first stitch stopped the bleeding almost instantly; the patient immediately improved. Had matters gone otherwise, there would have been a live infant with a deceased mother.

The second instance that I will never forget happened just days before intrauterine surgery, or surgery within the uterus, was possible for the patient. Thank goodness this time the patient had an experienced obstetrical physician. The patient's fetus had severe hydrocephalus, meaning the head of the fetus was extremely enlarged with a dangerous amount of excess fluid accumulation. Indeed, the head was so large that it could not fit through the birth canal in a normal manner. It was, however, pointed down toward the pelvis. The experienced obstetrical physician consulted with another ob/gyn specialist, and they agreed that the situation was hopeless as far as the baby was concerned. The degree of brain damage was severe, and no good therapy for this was available.

Eventually, after consult and discussion with the patient and her husband, the decision was made to do a procedure to collapse the skull and deliver the baby through the birth canal avoiding a Cesarean section. I suppose with present surgical advancements, the decision might now favor a Cesarean section. However, as I recall, this was the woman's first pregnancy, and doing so would have made it highly unlikely that she could ever deliver vaginally again if she became pregnant.

I will never forget the absolutely horrendous silence as the procedure went forward.

The patient was given anesthesia and the cervix was dilated. An instrument was then inserted and the skull collapsed. Extraction of the fetus was then performed. It is completely impossible to describe the feelings of morbidity, solemnity, and despair that filled that room. The two nurses and the attending physician performing the procedure as well as the two residents and myself were absolutely silent. There was simply nothing, nothing at all to say. A human life was being deliberately terminated.

This experience stood in total contradistinction from the usual happy, congenial attitude that was present in all of us when delivering live babies. I learned that day that regardless of one's philosophy or religious opinions, absolute awe is the universal emotion when faced with causing the death of a human being. This is true even when done deliberately and with forethought and mercy.

There was no question that the decision that was made in this instance was appropriate to the time and place. Yet to this day, some sixty years later, I still remember the feeling of despair and hopelessness that I shared with everyone in that room. This feeling lasted for many hours after, permeated our souls, and remains with me even now.

Chapter Ten

Physical Diagnosis

THE CLINICAL YEARS were those in which a resident actually dealt with patents on a one-to-one basis daily. These were the third and fourth years of medical school. Most of the instruction took place in a hospital or clinic setting. I learned physical diagnosis, along with three of my classmates, by being sent to Hines Veterans Hospital in a suburb of Chicago.

Each Saturday morning, the four of us met there with the senior instructor who was the chief resident in Internal Medicine. He started with the proper way to take a history, and proceeded with how to do a physical examination. The course ran for nine calendar months—an intensive training in the use of our hands, ears, eyes, nose, and other senses in evaluating patients' physical bodily functions.

Our instructor was a jovial, even-tempered, and patient Czech gentleman named Dr. Kobenz. After several weeks, however, I became isolated from the other three students in the group—not physically but isolated seemingly by the results of each morning's work.

Our day started by examining a patient and say describing a heart murmur. We all knew what we were supposed to hear in such a situation; the instructor had already told us what we would hear. We had also read about such situations in the textbook. Given the symptomatology and the physical findings presented, one of us would then come up with an appropriate physical or structural diagnosis. This continued every Saturday for nine months. However, I did not always hear or find what the other three did.

Finally, on the last day of the semester, Dr. Kobenz, with his usual affirmative smile, announced we were to go to a certain dark exam room and examine the right eye of the patient found there. We were not to ask the patient any questions—we were only to examine the eye and then describe what we saw in the *fundus*, or back, of the eye. Dr. Kobenz's final comment was that the patient was a chronic, hypertensive, black diabetic in renal failure.

All three of my contemporaries went into the room and came back out, each expounding on the details of the patient's diabetic hypertensive retinopathy and the pathological changes they had observed in the eye, such as retinal arteriouvenous nicking, or AV nicking; changes in light reflections; hemorrhages; and exudates, a mass of cells and fluid seeping from the blood vessels. Dr. Warner then chimed in with his usual other-worldly description of what he had seen. Finally, true to form for the last nine months, I gave my observations—my completely different observation: I simply could not see anything at all!

It wasn't that I hadn't tried. I had made every effort to examine the patient's right eye for problems, but could see nothing of any value in that regard.

And then, a miracle!

"You are correct, Warner!" Dr. Kobenz declared. "The patient has an artificial eye; you can see absolutely nothing inside this eye."

I was vindicated!

My three contemporaries, however, were exposed. They had lied about what they had seen that day. In fact, they had been simply parroting the descriptions given by Dr. Kobenz the entire nine months. With my contrary performance each and every Saturday morning, I ended the term with an A+; each of them, with a D-.

The wonder is that the four of us stayed amiable, or at least on speaking terms.

Chapter Eleven

Dr. Mark

UNDOUBTEDLY, ONE of our most interesting professors was Donald K. Mark. A rotund, outspoken, knowledgeable (and proud of it) import from Great Britain, Dr. Mark was known for quoting at length from obscure medical journals published in far-flung places such as South Africa, Hong Kong, and the like.

I will never forget one presentation of his that featured a thin elderly man in a wheelchair. This gentleman spoke with a distinct European accent, and was obviously a member of Chicago's famous immigrant culture, as was I. After the residents and others had asked their questions, the unanimous conclusion was that the gentleman was malnourished. Specifically, as Dr. Mark explained, because he did not eat American hamburgers, steaks, chili, or other typical American carnivorous delicacies. This made him suspect for the diagnosis of malnutrition. However, when the audience question time came, mine was, "Are you, Czech?"

"Ya, ya," he answered.

I continued, "Good. Do you eat liver?"

The answer: "Ya, ya."

"Do you eat sweetbreads, pancreas, brains?"

He answered again, "Ya, ya."

I asked him if he ate kidneys and heart as in a stew?

His answer: "Ya, ya."

I asked him if he ate blood sausage, and the answer was again the same: "Ya, ya."

In other words, the answers to several simple questions (if you know what Czechs eat) had quickly revealed that the gentleman in question consumed an ample supply of protein of a high nutritional quality.

Dr. Mark was left apoplectic and scarlet before this august body representing Chicago's medical elite. I am pretty sure he never forgave or forgot me.

This could be because I later was a coconspirator with a brilliant senior resident named Dr. Alexander, to Dr. Mark's chagrin. Dr. Alexander was equally rotund, brilliant, and outgoing as his British counterpart but not nearly as impressed with himself. He and Dr. Mark were known for their epic fights over minute details of medical data; we often watched agog as they traded quotes from obscure medical journals to make their respective points. One day, Dr. Alexander gave Dr. Mark his comeuppance with a little help from me.

On that day, Dr. Mark was the consulting physician on the indigent ward, or what was then called *3 Upper*. The ward had twelve patients with curtains separating the beds. The routine consisted of a senior resident introducing an intern to present the individual case before the group. Then as the consulting physician, Dr. Mark followed up with some appropriate questions, an examination of the patient, and whether he agreed with the intern's diagnosis.

If needed, the resident was always available to provide more information, such as lab results, if asked. The process went on in an orderly way with patients one through eleven. Each time, Dr. Mark would interject with obscure quotes from medical journals and details from the physical examination. Meanwhile, Dr. Alexander participated in his amiable way until we arrived at the twelfth patient. The intern delivered his presentation, and Dr. Mark began to ask the patient questions.

His first was a doozy: "Madam, were you ever told that you had syphilis?"

Silence.

When he received no response, he pointed to the deformity in the tibia in her lower leg, which was syphilitic in nature, and said: "Gentlemen, I will tell you one thing. You can come up with a diagnosis if you will just use your eyes." The implication of this, of course, was that none of us had noticed the deformity—no matter how untrue.

Then in an arrogant, loud voice, he said to the patient, "What is your problem?"

Again, silence.

"Madam, when I speak, I am used to people answering me. I do not ask questions without a reason. Answer me!"

Silence.

Another blast of questioning brought only more silence. An observer might have noticed by then that the medical students had not only left but were outside in the hall laughing. This was true of the intern also.

At the foot of the bed (still not approaching her closely lest he be contaminated), Dr. Mark still stood. In a rage, he slapped the soles of the patient's feet, producing a resounding noise. Through laughter, Dr. Alexander was overheard to say, "Dr. Mark, you missed the diagnosis."

Dr. Mark looked astounded. "What diagnosis?"

"(The patient) has been dead for five hours, Dr. Mark."

There was nothing more to say.

Chapter Twelve

An Account of Three Deaths, Each Teaching Us a Lesson

THERE WOULD GO ON to be a trio of other telling cases that included the death of a brilliant fifty-year-old Chicago attorney at the top of his profession. He was brought into the emergency room unconscious with a fever of 105. A stiff neck was noted, and he was immediately admitted to our service. With the fever and change in mental status, it was assumed that the likely diagnosis would be meningitis.

When we obtained further history, though, the cause of his troubles became a little less clear. This included a recent history of difficulty at work. Historically known for finishing legal cases within a crisp time frame, he had begun to miss deadlines and to produce work that lacked his usual superb reasoning. He had also begun to make legal misjudgments. His office staff had noted that his normal meticulous attire had given over to poorly knotted and dirty ties, hanging askew from around his neck. He often left the top button of his shirt unbuttoned. His eating habits had become slovenly. He had been observed dipping his fingers into food and washing them off afterward in a glass of water. He appeared to have difficulty using utensils properly, a sign of behavior related to *apraxia*, or the loss of a previously learned complex motor behavior. The attorney's wife had noted that he had also become less caring, shorter tempered, and complained of severe headaches and nausea.

We had started our diagnosis without this additional history. As a result, in the beginning, we went about diagnosing meningitis. The first step to do this was to obtain spinal fluid for laboratory proof of the disease, and, secondly, to get a culture in order to obtain the appropriate bacteriological help as far as the most appropriate antibiotic to prescribe.

Meanwhile, by placing him on his side, we attempted to straighten his back as much as we could and proceeded with a spinal tap. Since I was the neurology resident, that was my task. The needle entered the spinal canal relatively easily, but immediately I realized that we had a major problem: Fluid began to spurt out. And the fluid appeared to be under high pressure. When we put the manometer on the spinal needle, the spinal fluid pressure read more than three hundred (twice the norm). The patient then abruptly gasped and stopped breathing. I realized that we had likely caused the posterior portion of his brain to herniate downward through the foramen magnum, the opening from the cranial vault proper to the spinal canal. This had caused respiratory arrest. I tried immediately to replace the fluid, but it was too late.

That gasp was, in fact, his last.

We had no difficulty obtaining autopsy permission from the family; they wanted to know what had happened too.

Later that afternoon, I finally received a page to come to Pathology. My first sight upon entering the autopsy room was a waxed board with the brain placed on it—a sight never to be forgotten.

The brain was studded with multiple quarter- to half-inch nodules that appeared fleshy in nature. Under the microscope they revealed themselves to be metastatic melanoma. Melanomas are usually highly invasive, extremely malignant, and, in those days, totally unresponsive to treatment. Hence, the attorney's demise had probably been inevitable. Nonetheless, it was my putting the needle into his lumbar spine in an attempt to secure the diagnosis that had caused his death.

This case raised the challenge that all physicians understand: first, do no harm.

As we approach a patient, this is the basis for all diagnostic and therapeutic maneuvers in medicine that follow. In the case of the brilliant lawyer, we had not only done harm, we had precipitated his death.

All these years later, I have not forgotten this.

* * * * *

The second telling case was that of a thirty-five-year-old, previously healthy black mother of five who visited the clinic. Her history was that of progressive difficulty with balance and gait, headache, a decrease in level of consciousness and attentiveness, and a change in personality. I noted all of this along with the five little stair-step children that her husband brought along to the clinic.

We admitted her to the hospital and did the usual laboratory evaluation for a new patient. There was no more history to be obtained except that which we had obtained, and her laboratory work—that is, the usual initial laboratory work—was normal. A spinal tap, however, revealed spinal fluid with *pleocytosis*, basically an increased number of white blood cells. This indicated probable infection or at least inflammation. The protein level was also high, and the sugar was borderline low. These findings all suggested an infection. However, when we cultured the spinal fluid we could find no pathogens present. We looked for more exotic causes, such as a yeast infection or tuberculosis.

Again, nothing was conclusive.

This left me with a patient who had been gradually declining for no apparent reason. At this point, she had been seen not only by the medical students, the interns, and a junior resident but also by me—the senior neurology doctor on the house staff.

When in doubt—when looking at a probable bad result or when you don't have an answer, a thinking doctor always asks for consultations. The family readily agreed to this, and consultations were obtained from my immediate professor of Neurology and the chief of Neuropsychiatry.

The latter was an extremely gifted clinician by the name of Dr. Lauren Avery. Dr. Avery was among many of the great names in neurology and was considered an expert in his field. Suggestions from both of these two individuals were promptly followed but all proved to be no help in making the diagnosis.

I reached out to several other professors, including those in the areas of infectious disease and internal medicine. These were the teaching experts from the university hospital and medical school. Again several suggestions were made, but none of these consultations gave us a diagnosis, and because there was no diagnosis, no treatment was started.

This woman was dying in front of our eyes in one of the best hospitals in the greater Chicago area with multiple consultations at the highest level. Still, we were without a diagnosis. All anyone could think about was this mother not being at home to take care of her five children, when we weren't thinking about the husband who might be left to raise those five children on his own. In the end, she died, and then the same scenario I had experienced with the lawyer repeated itself.

Later in the day, I was paged to come to the pathology laboratory. There being no pagers or cell phones, I heard only a constant overhead request echoing throughout the hospital, "Calling Dr. Warner, calling Dr. Warner—report to Pathology."

Once again, I walked in to an unfixed brain on a waxed board at the end of the table. Once again, the brain was studded with miliary nodules; only this time, they proved to be *miliary tuberculosis*. Why this did not evidence itself in the spinal fluid studies, no one could explain.

Despite the best consultations and care available at the time, a positive diagnosis had not been made for this patient. As a result, appropriate therapeutic measures had not, and could not, be taken, and the patient died despite there being a treatment for what had ailed her. Even in 1959, we had a treatment for tuberculosis if we could only have proved that was what she had, if only we could have made the diagnosis.

* * * * *

The last of our three cases was a that of a fifty-five-year-old man with severe rheumatic valvular heart disease. He had had rheumatic fever as a child and had severely scarred heart valves that were causing obstruction of the outflow of blood from the heart as a result. This can produce heart failure after a period of compensation. Basically, the patient was slowly dying of overt congestive heart failure. The treatment would be open heart surgery, which, in those days, was a pioneering adventure but could improve or correct such a valvular problem.

After he underwent heart surgery, the senior surgical resident and I were left as the attending house staff, supervised by the attending surgical staff and medical/neurology staff. From the legal standpoint, the patient was the senior staff's responsibility. From the practical standpoint, everyday and night care of the patient was ours.

I well remember what a night that was.

Following the long day before, we spent the entire night drinking coffee and trying to decide what to do as we watched his blood pressures descend incrementally and his heart rate gradually rise. He became slowly more obtunded and less responsive. Like the others, he appeared to be dying before our eyes.

To make matters worse psychologically for us, his family members were there—witnessing all of this and asking if something more could be done for him. Multiple telephone calls went back and forth with the attending staff.

No one had any idea what else to do.

As the night came to an end, the effort to make a diagnosis fell to the surgical resident and me. We tried everything we knew to decipher the problem, yet the patient gradually faded away and finally died.

Over the next several days, we had multiple meetings of a soul-searching variety. We spoke with the attending staff and to basically anyone else who might have any knowledge as to what could have gone so wrong. We went over all the laboratory work in detail and reviewed all of the testing. We also evaluated what other procedures could have been done. Still, at the end of the day, no one had any new answers.

The autopsy would state that he died of gradual depletion of his blood volume.

This was not the complete answer but the only answer that we, or the family, would get. In this case, the patient died without any direct intervention of physicians—and without a satisfying cause ever being identified or proven at the autopsy afterward.

If one considers all three of these cases, important lessons emerge. We learned that no matter how careful, thoughtful, and meticulous a doctor might be, patients will die under our care.

After the death of the second patient, the mother of five, I went into a deep depression. Having been the one most personally involved in her care, I felt a high level of responsibility for her death. After three days of depression, during which I continued to function as a physician, Dr. Avery asked me, "What in the blazes is wrong with you, Warner?" I reminded him about the case. He had seen the patient in consultation and remembered her.

In response, he simply looked at me and asked, "Did you do everything you knew how to do?"

"Yes."

"Did you leave anything undone that you wish you would have done?"

My answer, "No."

"Did you get consultants to cover other possibilities?"

"Yes."

With that, he said: "When you have done everything you can, there is no more to be done. You are not responsible for the patient's death in any way."

What a relief to have someone—especially an authoritative, extremely kind, and committed physician—give me that reassurance. It was something I most certainly needed at that stage of my medical career.

In the end, these three cases teach the lesson that the public sometimes has great difficulty comprehending: no matter how far you go with medical care, there is a certain point at which you might hit a wall.

This was true then, and even with imaging, immunotherapy for cancer, and other new technology, this remains true still.

The existence of cases in which all therapy fails and no clear diagnosis ever appears remains. The physician must deal with the internal struggle that arises from this for the rest of his or her life. Such losses, when they come, remain permanent memories. In my opinion, this is probably why physicians often have a rather closed society in the sense that they tend to have few close friends; tend to be loners; and most friends are usually other physicians.

The opposite type of physician does exist here and there, but most of the physicians whom I have known through more than six decades are individuals who have lived within their own frame of medical knowledge. Perhaps this is the reason why physician suicide is relatively common, as is depression and burnout.

Chapter Thirteen

Dr. Maples

ONE OF THE MORE INTERESTING characters in Chicago was Dr. Maples, the Chief of Medicine for the hospital. A brilliant and talented physician and administrator, he demanded perfection from all of his residents. Each day at 1300 hours (1:00 p.m.), we would meet in his office to report on the new cases that had come in overnight to the hospital. This gave us an opportunity to discuss problems that we might have encountered with the Chief. It was always a most enlightening and challenging gathering.

One Friday afternoon, we arrived to find that a crisis had developed in the hospital the previous night involving a critical (and politically well-placed) patient. Dr. Maples knew this patient extremely well. Unfortunately, he also knew that the case had been mismanaged by one of my fellow residents. The data the resident handling the case had obtained had led him down the wrong path of diagnosis, and the patient had not fared well because of it.

By the next day, Dr. Maples was aware of the mistake and livid as a result. As he reviewed the case with the residents, he asked which of them was responsible. When nobody raised a hand, he became furious and demanded again to know who was responsible—we all knew that said person would be severely punished and probably kicked out of residency. To be kicked out of residency at this hospital was akin to committing medical suicide.

Having discussed the case with the other senior resident, I knew all of the facts involved. It was quite clear that if the facts surfaced, they would not be well tolerated. Punishment would be meted out for the outcome, rather than any failure of judgment. Failure of judgment was, of course, common to each and every one of us sitting in that room, as we well knew.

Nonetheless, Dr. Maples did not relent.

Instead, he stood up from his desk and began to rant and rave, profanity spewing in a torrent. We had never seen this brilliant man act in such a manner and were both shocked and perplexed. Trying to discuss anything at that point with him would have been like trying to reason with a raging bull. As I noted, I knew all the facts, but fortunately Dr. Maples didn't know that I was aware of them.

Finally, the session ended, and the residents filed out of the room, leaving me alone with Dr. Maples, a man I knew was the son of a clergyman.

"Dr. Maples," I said, "your father would not have appreciated his son's using language such as you have been today."

I then turned my back on him and walked out.

Thinking back now, I realize my behavior that afternoon showed a remarkable lack of insight into what could have happened to me (not to mention my medical career) that day. I prefer to believe that it also took a great deal of courage on my part to confront such an inappropriately angry Chief of Medicine.

The issue was never mentioned again by him or by me, and no further discussion was ever held regarding it.

Chapter Fourteen

Personal Episodes

A WEALTHY WOMAN, WHOM we will call The Dowager, lived in an opulent mansion filled with antiques in Oklahoma City in an elegant part of town. She became a patient of mine and, for some reason, became very fond of me as an individual as well as a physician. She had a full-time maid, a valet (as well as a husband), and several other house servants.

She was extremely wealthy.

She also was extremely arrogant and demanding. The word that comes to mind to describe her and her attitude toward others (excluding me) would be *imperial*. She ordered her husband around as if he were a puppy, and her tone with her hired help always carried an air of superiority and disdain.

I remember one day receiving a frantic call from The Dowager to come to her aid. Since there was no real ambulance service at the time (patients were transported in hearses from local funeral homes), I agreed to come immediately to address the emergency.

I arrived to find she had fractured a hip.

The diagnosis was easy—the extrication of the patient from her circumstances, more difficult. To paint a picture, The Dowager had slipped under her vehicle and was now stuck halfway between the front and back axles with nothing but her head and neck visible to me. She appeared to be in extreme pain. The pain, however, had not diminished her capability to order people around, which she was doing as I arrived. Her valet was running around like a madman, and her son and daughter were wailing like a Greek chorus. I ordered the valet to call the best ambulance service available and told her children to hush as they were disturbing both the patient and me. I then asked for the keys to the car.

By the time the ambulance arrived twenty minutes later, I had given The Dowager a shot of morphine and her screaming had decreased. I had also slowly moved the vehicle back enough to gain a few inches to the left and right of her. She was now fully exposed, so someone was able to put an appropriate appliance on her leg to stabilize it, move her onto a stretcher, and take her to the hospital for orthopedic care.

This unfortunate episode appeared to firmly bond me to The Dowager as her physician. I suspected this new allegiance was due in part to my seemingly being the only person who would stand up to her without worrying about the consequences.

Over the course of The Dowager's recovery, I was also made aware that she had a lovely granddaughter who resided in one of the larger cities in the eastern United States. When said granddaughter made a visit to the hospital, I introduced myself. She was a delightful, attractive, unmarried twenty-two-year-old, which seemed to be of concern to her entire family—especially her grandmother.

As I got to know The Dowager's granddaughter, I soon realized she was the only one in the family who had any sense. This was an important discovery given that I had come to realize her grandmother was going to need further care, and we would need a responsible adult to help make decisions about that care.

I had come to this conclusion as The Dowager's son continued to be reduced to whimpering in the presence of his mother while her timid daughter appeared to be totally under her control. I decided to see if the granddaughter might be up for the responsibility.

Having made it a practice to never dine alone with a woman who was not my wife, I invited The Dowager's granddaughter to lunch with Mrs. Warner and myself, and the three of us had a delightful time. At the close of lunch, we all said goodbye and separated amiably.

Weeks later, after The Dowager was back recovering at home, I received a phone call that she was in need of a house call. Usually such a call would stem from a complaint to be addressed, and the discretion of how to address the issue left to the physician, but not with The Dowager. I inquired as to the nature of the problem and was relayed to the maid, who said it could not be solved nor discussed on the telephone. I replied that I would come in the afternoon.

Upon my arrival, The Dowager ordered the maid to bring me a coffee; it arrived in a beautiful porcelain cup. As I sipped it, The Dowager ordered the maid to leave the room and shut the door behind her. This was unusual, as most patients want other people around to hear what the doctor has to say, if only so they can reiterate it at a later date. I was intrigued.

Once alone, The Dowager said in so many words, "Doctor, I know you well, and I admire you a good bit."

So far, so good.

"Do you know that I am a rich woman—*very rich?*"

"Well, yes, of course," I said, thinking about all of the property I had learned she owned around town as well as the many oil wells.

"Are you aware that whoever marries my granddaughter will get all of this money?"

"No," I replied, "that is none of my business, actually."

"You are a good man. Why don't you marry my granddaughter? You will be a rich man."

I looked at her incredulously, wondering if I had heard her correctly. She then repeated what she had said again word for word. Essentially, if I would agree to marry her granddaughter, I would become rich.

I quickly pointed out, "You may not be aware, but I am married and have two children. Furthermore, I am *happily* married, and have no desire to marry anybody else."

The Dowager pursed her lips but continued to look at me, seemingly in deep thought. I continued to drink my coffee, admittedly fascinated by the conversation. After a few very long minutes, she said, "Well, I gather that you are not interested, at least at this time."

"That's correct," I said.

She replied, "Think about it, however, doctor. If you change your mind, let me know. This is a business deal, and anytime you want to take me up on the deal, I am still good for it."

I took this to mean that the offer would remain open should I ever wish to reconsider in the future. I thanked her and told her I appreciated the confidence that she appeared to have in me as a person. I am not sure what she thought of this—had she ever run into anyone that she was unable to persuade with threats or bribes.

Our business concluded, I returned home to tell my wife the story. She was not as amused by the events of my day as I was. I have not, as yet, ever told my children about The Dowager's offer. Some things children do not need to know about their parents.

* * * * *

While in medical school, many of us worked at emergency offices, blood banks, laboratories, and the like. This was Chicago, the heart of the Mafia world, and the school was in the inner city where mobsters, drug dealers, bookies and burglars, and other sorts of flotsam and jetsam of society dwelt.

At the close of my sophomore year, I had the opportunity to take over the job of one of the senior medical students who worked at an industrial surgeon's office on Lake Street in downtown Chicago. This was an interesting office in that it was a storefront but one with examination rooms and an X-ray room. Said X-ray room had absolutely no shielding, so when one took an X-ray, one received a dose of radiation. I dealt with this by buying a lead apron for myself.

In the back of the office, a doorway opened into the tavern next door. The idea was that one could walk next door, obtain a meal in the bar, and return to work without ever stepping outside the doctor's office. That was important because the neighborhood was in one of the city's worst crime areas. Directly above the office was a den for the distribution of narcotics—people raced up and down the outside stairways day and night. In such crime zones, there was a tradition that neither doctors nor nurses were to be hurt, so long as they were in whites. If they were dressed in civilian clothes, however, they were fair game.

This was the situation I had walked into. At night, we kept the door locked unless a patient was waiting outside. I slept on a pull-out, fold-up cot. Being an old building, the office was infested with cockroaches and large black water bugs. The water bugs were particularly difficult to tolerate because they would crawl across my face at night and wake me up.

However, I have found that when one needs a job, one will put up with almost anything—even bugs.

At least the water bugs didn't bite.

This is where I learned to suture under the tutelage of my friend who was about to graduate from medical school. In fact, I trace my proficiency in the area of suturing wounds, both traumatic and operative, to this job. The first case to come in was the usual bar-related head injury. I say *usual* because one of the classic ways that one gets injured in a bar fight is from the broken end of a beer bottle. Rotated back and forth into the scalp, it makes quite an effective weapon. I can also assure you that such lacerations bleed profusely. The fortunate part, of course, is that almost all of these patients are already under the influence of alcohol. If they are not agitated, the alcohol acts as a sedative. For someone who is just learning to suture and is apprehensive about doing so, it is helpful to have a patient sedated, even from alcohol.

My friend taught me to wash wounds out thoroughly and to trim the edges of the torn skin with a scissor. This is called debridement, and such a trim produces nice, fresh, tender tissue that makes it easier to sew the edges of the wound together. If the wound is deep, one places a double layer of sutures to close the tissue. In fact, I trace my proficiency in the art of suturing wounds, both traumatic and operative, to this job.

Late on another night, a call came in for help for someone at a nearby industrial plant. Wearing my white coat, I got into the clinic car and drove to what ended up being a huge paper mill. The noise and smell was incredible! One could not converse much less hear anything over the noise of the machines. The floor vibrated with their power. I found the patient lying alone in the middle of the floor with his knees pulled up, holding his abdomen with both hands. I tried to ask him what had happened, but all I could make out was, "I hurt, Doc; I hurt." I put my hand on his belly and immediately noticed that it was board-like, a classic physical characteristic of *peritonitis*. In this patient's case, he had perforated an ulcer. The care was a dose of morphine to decrease his pain so we could ship him off to the hospital, which I did.

* * * * *

One of the more interesting jobs of my medical career was in the office of an industrial surgeon at a steel factory near Gary, Indiana. In those days, open hearth furnaces, as well as Bessemer converters and blast furnaces, were common at such places. What was unusual was that the office had aspirin in six or seven colors. We would get a call at night that Blast Furnace Number Two had run out of pain pills for the workers, and they didn't want any other kind of pain pill but the purple ones! If we said we had run out of the purple pills, they would reply, "Nothing else works; they have to be purple!" Of course, all of the pills were the same—exactly the same product—just a five-grain aspirin tablet. However, the foreman of each furnace would insist that only one color worked, and we had to keep that in mind. I found this an amusing example of the placebo effect.

The factory was a huge but comfortable place to work, and the medical facilities were excellent. If I needed to see a patient in the field, I had my own driver to chauffeur me. I also had a nurse. The physician who ran the operation was an industrial surgeon. When I applied, he interviewed me at length about my previous education and work experience. Part of that interview consisted of the typical question, "Where did you go to college?"

When I said Wheaton College in Wheaton, Illinois, his response was, "Oh, so you are religious, I would suppose. Aren't you?"

"Religious? Yes, I guess you would classify me as that."

He replied, "Well, I don't think much of religious people, and I am not sure you would do a very good job."

I said, "Well, I don't know, but we can always try."

He looked at me for some time and then said, "Okay."

During the time I worked there, I had absolutely no problems with anybody or anything. It was a delightful experience. Unfortunately, the plant was also an hour and fifteen-minute drive in each direction—even on rapid transit. It was a lucrative position because I could work from Friday night until Monday morning and be paid for every hour. As I recall, we would get about sixty dollars for the whole weekend, which in those days was a lot of money!

When I finally left, the hiring physician made a point of calling me into his office and thanking me for my service. I was pleased by that.

He then looked at me and said, "You know, I understand that you are quite religious, but it doesn't seem to have made much difference. You worked out well, and you are a good physician."

I have to admit I mulled that declaration of confidence over in my mind quite a bit, and had to wonder what would have happened if I had made any significant mistakes!

* * * * *

Sometime after we moved to Oklahoma City in 1961, we became involved with Wycliffe Bible translators. A number of our friends had become translators, and we had helped support them. Part of Wycliffe's training of their recruits included having them first take a list of linguistics courses in the United States on the collegiate level. They had a training camp in southern Mexico, appropriately called Jungle Camp, where recruits were trained in how to survive in a third-world environment and keep themselves healthy and productive. I spent several tours at the camp teaching a basic medicine course.

As a baseline, almost every indigenous patient there had one or several varieties of intestinal worms. We had the capability of identifying the ova, or eggs, of worms under a microscope so we were able to treat them. Many of the patients also had *amebiasis,* which was chronic. Malaria was endemic in the area too, and some patients had malaria of a severe degree. When our family returned home, all of us— my wife, myself, and our two children—had worms; thankfully worms readily cleared with appropriate medication.

One day at the camp, a message came in by way of a runner: I was needed at the clinic right away! I arrived to find a mother holding a crying infant. A glance revealed the child had a markedly distorted left nostril, and both nostrils were discharging a copious amount of *purulent exudate,* or pus. A small amount of blood was also coming from the left one. The tissues were red, inflamed, and tender.

In the rural regions where coffee is raised, the coffee beans, after ripening, are put out to dry. After they dry, they shrink in size and are then roasted and processed. This child had put one of the dried coffee beans up his left nostril—proving as anyone who has raised children knows full well that children the world over often delight in putting objects into their mouths, noses, ears, and such. In this instance, the bean had resided in the nostril for some days and would not budge. The tissue had become swollen and was grossly infected.

I had, of course, never seen such a thing. Nevertheless, I followed the basic tenets that I had learned in my internship in Ear, Nose, and Throat medicine. Nose drops, or *neosynephrine*, compliments of one of the campers were repeatedly applied to the child's nostril, causing the tissue to shrink. We then swaddled the child so that he could not move and asked his mother to hold him firmly.

A previous team had left behind some dental instruments, including a shaft with a ninety-degree hook at the end. The hook itself was about one-quarter-inch long. By this time, the mucosa had somewhat shrunken in the nose so we had a little room to work with. However, I could still only see the distal end of the coffee bean.

It was time to act. I inserted the probe along the upper surface of the bean. When I thought I had reached the back of it, I rotated the instrument ninety degrees and then gently pulled on it. Thanks to the lubrication provided by the abundant mucous, the bean popped out like a Jack-in-the-Box. Everyone was delighted. The little boy left with a prescription for antibiotics, and he had an uneventful recovery. Score one for basic medical training!

Over time, we took some teenagers (and later, adults) to the camp. Given the planes used to make the trip, we had to puzzle together passengers by weight. Despite our senior minister alone weighing in at more than a hundred kilos, we managed to get everyone placed on the Mission Aviation Fellowship plane and flown into camp.

A five-day walk from the nearest town, the camp had no roads, no refrigeration, and no flush toilets. It was our base for teaching the trainees medicine while also taking time to explore the area. I still remember taking the trainees on a canoe trip that had us pulling the canoes up the shallow river and then shooting the rapids coming back down. Our senior minister's enthusiasm for the process was more akin to that of an eighteen-year-old than a man in his fifties. At one point, I warned him to go slowly because he was no longer eighteen.

"Don't be in such a hurry!" I advised.

He was having too much fun to listen, and then he collapsed in the water! It took several of us to pull him back into the canoe. I sent my wife with the rest of the women upstream; the last thing I needed was several women screaming or praying over the pastor, who in their defense, did look as though he were dying.

With them gone, we moved downstream a short distance and rolled his body out on some flat rocks. He remained unresponsive, and by now, his body felt cold and clammy. He was also short of breath. I swam up the river to where a group of male campers were bathing and requested that they immediately run up to Jungle Camp (about a hundred yards up a narrow path to the gorge where the river began) and obtain a stretcher. They returned with an Army stretcher from World War II; we rolled the minister onto it and carried him back up the hill. That was quite a chore because, remember, he weighed more than 100 kilos—or two hundred and twenty-plus pounds.

The narrow path was such that Americans had to stagger up it with their feet apart, while the indigenous locals walked it with one foot right ahead of the other. To carry the stretcher uphill on such a slippery, narrow trail was a feat. When they got the minister uphill, the nurse trainees pitched right in. Fortunately, I had added some morphine sulfate to the medicine cabinet on a previous trip. I gave the minister one dose, and later another. By the time the mission plane returned, the patient was responsive and no longer *dyspneic* (short of breath). However, he still exhibited less than his normal alertness and cognition.

We put him on the plane along with a nurse, and flew out to Altamirano, a small Catholic mission hospital. As the single-engine plane circled Jungle Camp, gaining altitude slowly, we looked down and saw the campers standing in a circle, holding hands, and praying—we could only assume for a safe trip for the minister and the rest of us.

In the end, all ended well.

In a few days, the minister was back in the States undergoing further medical evaluation. His preaching was not adversely affected by his experience. Later, my wife told me that the gentleman who ran the camp had asked, " 'Doesn't he (meaning me) ever get excited when something goes wrong?' "

" 'No,' " she said she told him. " 'The only time he gets excited is when he loses something!' "

Such is the insight of a wife who has been married for a long time.

We later had a similar experience with a Mexican anesthesiologist who had trained in the States. While having lunch with him at a local ranch, I went to get more food (*superb* Mexican food, which I *dearly* love), while my wife continued her conversation with the anesthesiologist, who spoke fluent English.

" 'I'll bet that he is the one in a medical emergency or disaster who stays perfectly calm,' " he told her.

My wife said she replied, " 'Yes, absolutely.' "

I confess that I have never understood how becoming

excited and losing control of your emotions made any situation better.

* * * * *

Back in Chicago, while I was in medical school, my wife integrated a one-city-block-square, four-story-high inner city school there. In 1956, she was one of two white teachers in this massive school, along with the principal. Everyone else was black.

Both the building we lived in and the school itself have long since been dismantled, but at the time, the school was teeming with students. My wife taught a large class and was determined to help as many of the children in her charge as she could, as many ways as she could. I shouldn't have been surprised when I got a telephone call from her after school hours saying, "We need to go to see one of my students."

The young man was in jail, and while I wouldn't normally make police station calls in Chicago in my medical whites, I knew better than to argue. We drove our old jalopy down to the police station to find my wife's student.

Michael (not his real name) had stolen a jacket and then attempted to sell it. He had been picked up by the police and was facing charges. Hunger, rather than greed, had motivated his actions. He had stolen the jacket to sell for money so he could buy food. Michael had refused to go into the drug trade, which was the way many people in his neighborhood made money. His mother was a prostitute, and she did not feed him.

The child was starving.

Upon learning this, without any further discussion, I said to the police officer, "We will be responsible for him."

This agreement would mean that the police no longer needed to be concerned about the boy, while Michael gained a safe haven with three squares a day and a place to lay his head.

"Of course, Doc," the officer replied. "If you want to be responsible for him, that would be great."

And so we did. Michael came to us from the kind of deprived background that makes for tragic after-school TV specials. We believed he had been sent to us for us to help, but I knew some boundaries needed to be drawn right away if this was going to work. I bluntly told him, "Michael, we will give you food, clothes, a place to sleep, but we will not give you money."

We followed through on our promise.

Michael went on to finish school, earn his plumbing license, and become gainfully employed in Chicago. He later visited us several times in Oklahoma before we lost track of him. The moral of this story: It is better to light one candle than to curse the darkness. In Michael's case, we were given the opportunity to be of assistance to this one individual, and we took it—resulting in a good outcome for all of us. Years later while visiting us in Oklahoma, Michael would tell us, "Every boy in my class is dead or in jail except me."

One young life had been saved, but sadly, many others were lost.

* * * * *

I was trained in bioethics by a Jesuit. I took the course in Berkeley, California. We worked many hours a day in the program, learning how to run an ethics committee while also learning basic bioethics.

Back in Oklahoma City, I organized a bioethics committee based on what I had learned. When I returned to California six months later to report to my mentor on my progress, I waited for everyone else to finish and depart before I spoke with him. I had gone so far as to arrange a red-eye flight home so that I could stay later with my mentor to address some things that had been bothering me.

After the room cleared, I said to him, "John, I understand the mechanisms of creating an ethics committee and the idea of a common consensus on a case. However, you have not taught the important part: that ethics come from God and the scriptures and the concept of 'man being made in the image of God' as the foundation of all of our understanding of human values."

He looked at me somewhat amused and said, "Ernie, don't you realize that the rest of them haven't even started to ask those questions?"

Well, obviously I had not.

I left still convinced that the underlying *reason* for bioethics was as important for doctors to know and understand as its practical application. For me, bioethics training was like a theological program that flows over into the practical aspects of our daily life . . . and how we live it.

Chapter Fifteen

Fecal Impaction

ECAL IMPACTION. The first time I heard these words, I was innocently unaware of this dreaded diagnosis. That soon changed as the responsibility of removing a fecal impaction case fell to me, the intern—the lowest member on the medical staff totem pole.

Fecal impaction is the medical term for a mass of feces that has stayed in the rectum long enough to have turned into an almost solid object. This results in an obstruction of the flow of fecal matter outward, creating something like a dam that must be removed manually—that is, by hand—and in this case, by my hand!

I grasped the extraction process but very much wished someone else could step in to do it in my place. And, yes, standard procedure was to lubricate the index finger and insert the finger into the rectum until the hard mass was palpable or able to be touched. The mass was then broken up digitally—that is, by finger pressure—into smaller pieces and extracted.

In this instance, the first extraction of feces caused a wave of severe nausea followed by retching—not in the patient but in the extractor. The stool had been stalled for six or seven days by that point, and the odor that came with its removal was awful!

Nonetheless, continue the procedure I did.

After the full mass was removed, the patient was more than grateful, and henceforth, when I was in charge of a rehabilitation unit, I made a point never to let this happen to a patient.

Yes, *fecal impaction can be avoided.*

The secret is to meticulously observe and record all patient bowel movements. In some cases, the patient is placed on stool softeners or mild laxatives, such as Senna, which I have found produces good results in virtually all patients. Thank goodness for laxatives! Thank goodness for stool softeners and for rubber gloves.

That said, I would argue every young physician should perform a fecal impaction removal at least once—a sure fire way to ensure that the doctor never forgets the possibility of bowel obstruction or impaction in the future.

Chapter Sixteen

Obtaining Autopsy Permissions

IN MY DAY, ONE OF THE major tasks of the hospital house staff was to obtain permissions for autopsies from the family or next of kin of the deceased. This was extremely important work because the authorities rated the hospital partially on the basis of its autopsy rate.

As I recall, the hospital needed to obtain an autopsy rate of about 85 to 90 percent to keep a respectable rating. Today, this rate has fallen to about 5 percent. Yet even in my time, getting permission was difficult because most grieving families are not in the mood to talk about an autopsy if they already have a probable diagnosis of what caused their loved one's death. In the absence of our present-day imaging and extremely accurate, well-tuned diagnostic studies, though an autopsy was the only way to monitor quality in medical care in the hospital setting. Hence, the insistence on a high autopsy percentage of our deceased patients.

In Chicago, a large number of Italian-American patients lived in the community within the immediate vicinity of the hospital. Many of them ended up as patients who subsequently died. Most of the Italian families we served were large families; they would often have five, six, or more children spread around the various parts of the city as well as outside of the Chicago area. Autopsy permission had to be obtained from *all* of these persons to be considered legitimate.

I remember one deceased mother who had six children. The first two were present when she died, and after some cajoling and discussion, they gave permission for the autopsy to be done. An hour passed and another relative appeared who had to give permission. Again, there was much crying, moaning, and screaming as well as more discussion about the wonderful attributes of the recently deceased and how she would be missed by her children, grandchildren, and community. This ritual took about an hour before the new visitor was ready to be approached and permission obtained.

Indeed, the family was so large that over the next several hours, new members continued to appear one by one, with each newcomer being offered condolences by the house staff. Each arrival triggered a replay of this grief ritual as well as our efforts to get the latest newcomer's permission for the autopsy.

The stress on the house staff grew as the hours passed, many, many hours. Obtaining permissions in such situations is something of a fine art, one developed by the residents to make certain an autopsy for every patient who expired in our hospital was secured. Rarely did we end up without permission. This, in fact, is a direct demonstration of the confidence these patients and their families had in the history and quality of medical care at this landmark Chicago hospital.

Chapter Seventeen

Anesthesia

IN THE FIRST YEAR after graduation from medical school, my peers and I entered the *internship*. I ended up on anesthesia service for two months. This proved to be a great time of learning and gaining experience as anesthesiology is a demanding medical specialty—one that requires quick, difficult decisions.

During surgery, one of the major ways that the airway of a patient is controlled—that is, how a physician ensures a patient is adequately ventilated while unconscious—is by inserting an endotracheal tube. These tubes are made in various sizes and types for individual patients. They are inserted by placing a laryngoscope, an L-shaped instrument, into the mouth and throat and depressing the tongue so that the larynx or voice box can be seen before insertion for clear placement. In my experience, when the tube was finally inserted, we would blow into it to make sure that both sides of the chest inflated—not just one. If both sides inflated, the tube was assumed to have been successfully inserted and was then connected to an anesthesia machine. The catch, of course, was how to learn to do intubation on live patients in a safe manner.

After considerable thought, I came up with the ingenious idea of practicing intubation on the recently deceased. Since I was well known to all of the house staff having taken the last two years of my medical studies at the hospital, our trust in each other and communication was superb. From that point on, when a patient was soon to die, someone would call to say a death was imminent. I would then put some endotracheal tubes in one white coat pocket and a laryngoscope in the other and wait for death to occur.

As soon as the patient expired, the family would go into the usual autopsy discussion at the end of the corridor in a consultation room with the house staff. Meanwhile, I would head to the recently deceased's room to practice intubating while the patient's body was still supple, and often warm.

This may sound macabre to a lay person, and perhaps in this time of rights and litigation unwise, both morally and legally. Of course, that begs the question, *How does one learn to do a process to save the lives of multiple patients without ever having a patient to practice on?*

My solution to this problem may not have been perfect, but it did work. I became adept at intubating patients, which I like to think benefited my future patients. As I progressed and the Chief of Anesthesia, Dr. Middleton, became more confident in my ability to anesthetize patients, I was given more liberty to take charge of the process during surgery. As I recall, the first time I was left alone with a patient (without Dr. Middleton or another senior anesthesiologist supervising me), I was *terrified*!

I still remember inserting the needle and injecting the patient with sodium pentothal. With the unconscious patient no longer breathing, I had only a brief moment to intubate. I extended the neck in the proper manner and inserted the laryngoscope only to realize I had an obstructed view through it. I simply could not observe the larynx well enough to take the next step.

Finally, with a quick repositioning of the neck (the patient was still not breathing), I was able to clearly see the larynx and insert the tube. I puffed rapidly into it and watched the chest inflate several times, on both sides. With that, I hooked the patient up to the anesthesia machine, and all was well.

Throughout this entire process, I was alone in the cold, sterile operating room save for a scrub nurse setting up her instruments. To say that I gained confidence from the experience would be an understatement. Still, I remained concerned that I hadn't been properly supervised. I asked Dr. Middleton why he had left me to fend for myself despite this having been the first time for me to do the procedure on a live person.

He laughed vigorously and said, "You did great."

"How do you know that I did great?"

"Oh, I was watching you all the time," he said.

"Watching me all the time?"

"Yes, watching you all the time. I didn't miss a thing. You did great."

"I was terrified."

"Of course," he said.

"How did you watch me? I didn't see you."

"I was behind the door looking through the crack in the hinges, and could see you clearly. You were not in any trouble. Believe me, if you had been in trouble I would have been in there instantly."

His response left me dumbfounded.

What a lesson in pedagogical technique—let the student go as far as possible under unseen observation believing the procedure is being done without a parachute.

Yes, this is the way physicians learn—an experience that cannot be replicated by reading a book, or by watching a television or iPad screen. Technology can be of help, but hands-on experience is the only way to fully and effectively learn when you are a doctor.

Chapter Eighteen

General Medical Rotation

WE HAD A YOUNG WOMAN come into the hospital who was a known *myasthenic*. That is, she had myasthenia gravis. She went into a crisis and gradually began to lose the ability to breathe as we watched. In those days, no automated respirators existed. Instead, a doctor had to place an endotracheal tube before he or she could ventilate the patient with a bag or other device, alternating pressure to inflate the chest. On this day, we had tried to manipulate the young woman's medications but to no avail; she needed to be intubated.

We proceeded to do so, placing her on an anesthesia machine to breathe for her until a rather primitive mechanical respirator could take over the task. Thankfully, she slowly recovered with treatment.

The next Friday we presented her case at noon during Medical Grand Rounds. The audience that filled the amphitheater was comprised of our hospital peers but also medical personnel from nearby hospitals. The intern presented the case history, and the resident talked about the laboratory data along with other matters. My job as a neurology resident was to answer questions relative to the young woman's neurological care—in this case, the commentary was not all roses and platitudes.

Instead, one of the senior infectious disease attendees, a prominent female physician at one of the other hospitals, made a caustic comment to the effect that didn't this patient now have pneumonia too. This was true. The young woman was recovering well with antibiotics but had developed pneumonia.

The same professor then asked if when intubating the young woman, had a sterile endotracheal tube been used? And was the entire procedure done in an elective aseptic manner? I replied that no, hers had been an emergency intubation with the priority being to get her respirations under control in order to save her life.

The professor then said that in her opinion, the procedure should have waited until a sterile endotracheal tube could be procured, at which point the intubation should have been done under elective conditions. Her reasoning was that had these steps been taken, the young patient would not have developed pneumonia. I loudly retorted, "Well, it is possible that you are correct. However, in my opinion, it is better to have a live patient with pneumonia than a dead patient with a sterile airway."

This was greeted by absolute silence—and then by applause. My point had been made.

I did not make many friends as a result of some of my comments through the years, but for what it's worth, they were always spontaneous and genuine.

Chapter Nineteen

Diagnostic Pitfalls

W HILE IN GENERAL medical service, I once helped treat an elderly woman who had had a mastectomy for carcinoma of the right breast some sixteen years before. An enlarged lymph node under her right axilla, or armpit, had now brought her to us. Truth be told, the very idea that cancer could metastasize in the same node sixteen years later startled us all. However, the diagnosis was confirmed upon removal of the node. Her case raises questions about the prudence of using five- and ten-year survival data to prove efficacy of treatment.

In another case, a young woman came into the hospital emergency room with abdominal pain. The consensus of the five of us examining physicians was that she had appendicitis. The attending senior surgeon disagreed.

He believed she had contracted the polio virus. While it was summertime when the virus normally flourished, we took his diagnosis as a direct insult to our own. We made a wager—the five of us would treat the attending to a steak dinner if the young woman was found to have polio.

More tests and examination followed. We had progressed to a spinal tap when it became quite clear the patient had *pleocytosis*, an elevation of the white cells common with polio; she had also developed some other symptoms not present at the onset.

To this day, I still do not understand how the attending made his diagnosis so early—particularly given that he was a surgeon. Surgeons are generally known not for their diagnostic acumen but rather for their surgical skills. We later found out he had had experiences that we had not. He had also taught medicine earlier in his career in Lebanon—fortunately so for our patient, because if she had had abdominal surgery for appendicitis while suffering poliomyelitis, she might well have ended up paralyzed.

Despite the damage to our salaries, we five bought steaks and took them to the attending's house, thus paying off our lost bet over a nice meal.

The lesson of this story is that it often pays to listen to your more experienced elders!

Chapter Twenty

Subdural Hematoma

ONE OF THE MOST challenging cases I have ever encountered was one of my chief's. A woman from rural Illinois had fallen while leaving church one Sunday morning and hit the back of her head. Subsequently, she developed headaches, grew less attentive, and became lethargic. She was brought to the hospital, and her care fell to me and a young neurosurgeon.

The point of interest was to be found in her clinical course. There was no imaging in use at the time, and arteriograms (an imaging test that uses X-rays and a special dye to see inside the arteries) were available but extremely risky, as they were done by direct injection into the carotid artery in the neck. In other words, the diagnostic possibilities were limited, but the observational possibilities were endless. This is one of the problems with medicine today. Younger doctors rarely have the opportunity to observe illnesses developing in a time frame so that they can see the consequences of the illness and the pathological changes that ensue. On this particular day, time would tell.

While observing the patient, Dr. Monson, the neurosurgeon, noted that she had a weak right arm and a Babinski reflex—a neuro-pathological cue embedded within the plantar reflex of the foot—on her right side. The latter often a sign of a problem in the left cerebral hemisphere or the left side of the brain.

Dr. Monson called for me to reexamine the patient. I did as asked, but could find nothing wrong except her obtundation, or less than full alertness. The patient's skull X-rays were normal too, and the patient's EEG, or electroencephalogram scan of her brain waves, showed only nonspecific slowing. This prompted me to call the neurosurgeon and suggest that he might try learning how to do a proper neurological examination! (Friendly rivalry was a constant with our staff.)

Dr. Monson's next move was to reexamine the patient later that afternoon, only to report findings similar to his earlier ones. By the time I got there, of course, the signs were gone. He affirmed them again the following morning, but by the afternoon, when I returned, the symptoms once again no longer presented. To shorten the story, this pattern repeated itself over the next several days. The patient also demonstrated fluctuating neurological signs, which came and went, confusing us all. Nowadays, a simple CT scan or an MRI could likely solve such a problem in minutes. However, this was not an option in the 1950s.

Finally, we decided to do an arteriogram. The result this time was clear: The patient had bilateral subdural hematomas. A build up of blood was causing pressure on the surface of her brain. Hematomas usually occur on one side of the brain, but in this particular case, they were on both. With the patient being the chief neurologist's mother, maybe it was only fitting that she should have a perplexing neurological illness rather than heart disease or some more mundane diagnosis.

Dr. Monson commenced treatment, drilling small burr holes in both sides of the patient's head to remove both the blood and pressure. Sure enough, the patient woke up her old self, though I am sure going forward she was more careful where she placed her feet at church.

The lesson of this case is that some medical problems can only be resolved with the passage of time and the repeated examination and follow-up on one's findings. Again, this approach can be too often lost in the medical system of today—at least in the U.S. where medicine can feel as if it is being practiced with a stopwatch. Too many physicians are asked to make instantaneous diagnoses and to promptly treat the patient so the patient will *get well.* Unfortunately, TV medical dramas give people the same impression: solutions available within thirty minutes or less, an hour at the most.

This is not the way reality works, however.

Sometimes, as in the case of the mother of our hospital's chief neurologist, prolonged observation is necessary. I have found this to be particularly true in the case of psychiatric patients. Sometimes only after several days of observation of such a patient does the problem reveal itself— and the correct diagnosis become obvious.

Ideally, only *then* should treatment commence.

Chapter Twenty-One

Neurology Residency

O NE SATURDAY MORNING, a laborer came in the hospital complaining of balance issues after falling. He had weakness in all four extremities but with preservation of his face motion, eye motion, and consciousness. After taking his medical history, we learned that over the previous several weeks, he had gradually begun to stumble and lose his balance. He had also developed nausea and recurrent headaches.

The only neurosurgeon available that morning was a gifted but equally arrogant gentleman whom we will call Dr. Blade. Dr. Blade was known for insisting that his residents meet him each morning at the hospital door for rounds and for refusing to see a patient until a diagnosis was made that indicated a need for surgery.

In this case, Dr. Marvin did a myelogram, an imaging procedure that examines the relationship between your vertebrae and discs. This is a procedure that remains in use today. Basically, a radiopaque (X-ray opaque) contrast media is injected into the spinal canal, and then run up and down to see if any obstruction is encountered. In this case, an obvious obstruction in the neck was found, and it appeared to be a tumorous condition.

This occurred on a Saturday, and neurosurgeons don't like to operate on their days off, which is why this particular surgeon was the only one available. He came reluctantly to see the patient and decided that surgery was indicated on an emergency basis. The two neurosurgery residents took the patient to surgery, opened up the operative site to visualize the tumor, and the neurosurgeon came in to extricate it.

This took Dr. Marvin about two hours. The residents then closed up the wounds, and the patient was sent to recovery. The point of this story is that this patient was a manual laborer. The neurosurgeon sent him a bill for $5,000. Today, that bill would be, I would suppose, at least $50,000. Needless to say, the family was floored when it got the bill, particularly after learning that the tumor was malignant and no other treatment was available. The patient sadly would eventually die.

The family confided all of this to me, and I was perplexed as to how to handle the situation. Finally, I went to Dr. Marvin and said, "These are very poor people. They cannot afford $5,000. In fact, they will never see $5,000 at one time at any point in their lives!"

Dr. Marvin went to the neurosurgeon and asked if he could reduce his fee. The neurosurgeon did so by half ($2,500)—still a fortune for a laborer. Since the doctor was an extremely wealthy man, he could have reduced the fee to a token amount to preserve the family's dignity and finances. As the years went on, I recall many a time in my own practice when similar incidences occurred; I reduced the charges to a modicum—but not to zero! I believed then and I believe now that it is always important that patients pay something. Otherwise, what has been done for them may be seen as having no value at all.

* * * * *

One of the neurosurgical residents was a hunter from Colorado. He had a reputation as a crack shot and had brought his favorite rifle with him to Chicago. Like the rest of the residents, he parked his vehicle in the hospital parking lot, an open space with a chain-link fence around it. There was no guard nor other measures to protect our cars, or their contents, or us, for that matter. Since only physicians, residents, and such could park there, the lot was known to the neighborhood as the Physicians Parking Lot. As for the neighborhood itself, it was Mafia-controlled—from the grocery store, to the drugstore, to all other aspects of people's lives. Thankfully for us, the Mafia held physicians in high regard—hospitals too. This was mainly due to a belief that if anybody in the neighborhood were to be shot or otherwise injured, they would likely end up at one of the local hospitals for care. Hence the logic went, better to have local doctors as friends than not.

So peace reigned until the day the new Colorado resident witnessed a teen-aged boy from one of the Mafia families break into his car and steal some of its contents. The resident followed the boy home. After learning where the teen lived, he later returned to the house and knocked on the door. He asked the woman who answered, "Do you have a boy?" And he proceeded to describe the culprit.

"Yes, that's my son," she said.

The resident said, "Do you know your son is stealing from our cars over there in the parking lot?"

"My son would never do that," the woman said.

The resident replied, "Well, you defend him as much as you want to, but I saw him in our cars."

"That couldn't happen," she said.

"Well, it did happen. So let me tell you that I have a rifle and I am a crack shot. If that boy goes into that parking lot again, I will take him out. Do you understand that?"

"Yes, I understand that. Thank you," the woman said.

No one ever bothered another car in that lot. Sometimes direct action works, I suppose.

* * * * *

One night as an intern (that is, a first year postgraduate), I was on Ear, Nose, and Throat service and ENT emergency call. A patient came in with a nosebleed, or *epistaxis*, so severe he was bleeding out. I counseled with my attending physician, an ENT specialist, and he advised a Foley catheter (usually used for the urinary tract) be inserted in the nose. The balloon was inflated in the nasopharynx, and packing placed against it to stop the bleeding. It took some time, but we got the bleeding under control, and after several transfusions the patient was stable.

While the man was still bleeding acutely, he turned to me and said, "Here Doc, take care of this for me until I am well." He handed me a large roll of bills, about an inch and a half round, secured with rubber bands. I placed the wad of bills in the pocket of my white pants and promptly forgot about it.

The patient went on to be admitted. After another day or so, the attending physician carefully removed the packing in his nostrils and the catheter, and the patient was stabilized with no further bleeding. The man professed extreme gratitude for what we had done for him—basically saving him from bleeding out. Interestingly, no one came to see him. He had no visitors, no phone calls, no flowers, no nothing. As he was getting ready to leave, I handed back his roll of bills.

"Did you count it, Doc?"

"Of course not," I said, "I just stuck it in my pocket until you were ready to leave."

"You know, Doc, you saved my life. If you had not been here and stayed up with me all night and given me the blood, I probably would have died."

"Well, I suppose that's true, but that is our job."

He seemed to think about that for a moment, and then said, "Doc, I want to do you a favor."

With that, he reached into his pocket and took out a business card, which he handed to me. The card said:

Bill J. John Services, as needed

There was also a phone number (*again*, no cell phones in those days).

I looked at the card and said, "What will I do with this? What is it good for?"

"Well, Doc, I am in the business of rubbing people out. I'm good at it too, Doc. You saved my life, and I want to give something back to you as payment for what you have done for me, far beyond any money that may have changed hands."

I thought about it for a few minutes, looked at him, and said, "I gather what you say is you murder people on consignment."

He replied, "Yes, but I am good at it too, Doc."

He was obviously proud of his operation. I explained that I had no one who needed rubbed out, but would keep his card in the event that someday I might have need. I thanked him for his generosity and we said goodbye. Our exchange was just the way business was done back then in the Chicago underworld, and a good example of how the Mafia-made men treated physicians. They held us in high regard because their lives often depended on us.

* * * * *

The most fascinating and funny event of my internship year happened on Dr. Mel's watch. A general surgeon, he also did a good bit of abdominal surgery. So when a young woman came into the hospital with severe ulcerative colitis, it wasn't surprising that he was involved in her care.

At the time of this story, ulcerative colitis was an extremely difficult disease to treat; we had very few of the modern facilities and treatments available today, including even such simple measures as steroids. Instead, one of the go-to treatments was to do a colectomy. This called for the colon to be removed and an opening made in the abdomen that provided for the passage of liquid feces. Unfortunately, there is no valve involved in this situation, and so stool comes out repeatedly and in unpredictable quantities into a bag attached to the skin around the ileostomy opening.

On this day, our particular patient had had a colectomy and was several days postoperative. As we prepared to enter her hospital room, we heard peculiar sounds coming from it as we approached.

Usually our retinue proceeded strictly in order. The least important person entering first, followed by the next, with Dr. Mel, the chief, at the end. This day, however, for whatever reason, Dr. Mel walked in first.

The chief was a late middle-aged, somewhat portly, impeccably dressed surgeon. He traveled this day as he always did—in a well-tailored, three-piece suit with the vest buttoned; a gold watch chain across his ample abdomen;

and his tie carefully knotted. He walked into the woman's room, and before the rest of us could follow, screamed: "Come! Help! Help! Help!"

The resident and I barged into the room behind him, followed by the medical students—and burst into a paroxysmal fit of laughter. The elegant Dr. Mel had fallen into the embrace of a young naked woman, our patient who was still recovering from her recent colectomy. Multiple cups of liquid feces sprouted from her abdomen, their contents covering the front of Dr. Mel's three-piece suit, pouring into his shoes, and trickling down onto the floor. Dr. Mel was still crying for help, but we were all too amused by his predicament to assist at first. After a few moments, we rallied to the moment and attempted to separate the two of them—the patient and the surgeon—while also trying to avoid getting liquid feces all over us.

All was cleaned up, and ultimately, the patient was sedated. Eventually she went home. Many years have since passed, and I do not know if Dr. Mel remembers that day, but I surely do.

* * * * *

When it came to patient workups—that is patient evaluation—in neurology, routine blood work was the only lab test that all patients received. Besides that, neurological patients might have skull X-rays, an EEG, or a spinal fluid examination obtained by lumbar puncture. Skull X-rays were done to check for pineal gland displacement. Located in the middle of the cranium, the pineal gland can often become calcified. If so, the gland will show up displaced from its normal position on the X-ray by a tumor, a subdural hematoma, or some other mass. The electroencephalogram reveals the electrical activity of the brain. This is compared with the standard, or normal, values. Conclusions may be drawn by the frequency or the location of slowing, seizure activity and the like. The spinal fluid can be examined for evidence of increased pressure, infection, and inflammation, among other things.

These were not the only tools that we had in neurology, but were also the ones most commonly used on neurology patients. In problem cases, we could perform a carotid arteriogram, which entails puncturing the carotid artery in the neck and injecting a radio-contrast material. There would be rapid cassette changes, which flipped through a sequence of X-ray films, each one revealing the passage of the dye to the intracranial and extracranial circulation—*at least* the carotid circulation. The vertebral, or posterior, circulation, was less accurately imaged with this technique. Unfortunately, complications could occur, and they could be rather troublesome, particularly if repeated doses of dye were given.

Another invasive technique was that of *pneumoenceph-alography*, which involved placing a needle into the lumbar spine and taking a small sample of spinal fluid. Air was then injected with the spinal fluid being taken out at roughly the same proportional amount as the air being injected. The purpose of the air was to provide a contrast media. A tumor or mass could be outlined in silhouette against the injected air.

Displaying intracranial structures accurately remained difficult, but with a skilled operator, the images could be obtained. The air would be bubbled about the inside of the head as the body rotated in a spiral chair. Patients suffered severe 10/10 headaches and vomiting with the position. Compared to modern technology, this was primitive and certainly uncomfortable and risky for the patient.

In the present day with MRIs, CT scans, PET scans, and the use of intravenous contrast media to do such exams, it is a simple and virtually painless procedure. There is almost no risk of adverse effects. Unfortunately, the use of the new techniques, which are superb for diagnosis, have decreased the acuity of the physicians in many cases. For instance, with headaches, rather than following up with further questions as to frequency, location, length of time present, intensity, familial history, environmental factors, food choices, positional changes, sleep issues, and the like, physicians now leap immediately to imaging.

The cost, of course, is magnified by this type of reflex thinking. I recall a patient who was referred from the emergency room with no diagnosis except *neurological problems*. The patient had had an MRI scan of the lumbar spine, the dorsal (thoracic) spine, the cervical spine, and the head. None of these four studies, costing thousands of dollars at that time, gave the diagnosis. Instead, we needed to proceed by the standard methodology to complete the diagnosis. I find the automatic use of imaging techniques obviates the necessity for understanding the other problems that the patient might have, such as diabetes, hypertension, or hyperlipidemia.

When I teach residents, they will often start a case with a simple, one-sentence description of the patient and then go to imaging. They will see an abnormality on the imaging and blame the patient's symptoms on that. This is often not the case. That is, one might have migraine headaches, but one may also have uncontrolled diabetes, hypertension, or liver disease, which also must be addressed if the patient is to return to good health.

Chapter Twenty-Two

U.S. Army Medical Corps
July 1959 to July 1961

I SERVED IN THE U. S. Army Medical Corps as an internal medicine specialist with particular interest in neurology because that's the classification that fit me. I was stationed at Fort Campbell, Kentucky, from 3 July 1959 to midnight of 3 July 1961.

The transition from residence life to military life was abrupt but fascinating. And they paid me—eight hundred dollars per month compared to the hundred and seven dollars of my old job. The biggest jolt psychologically was the transition from the world of academic medicine and a residency program into the world of *real* medicine. For one, the number of patients increased geometrically. And if you were the officer of the day—you went on call from 0800 with no relief until the next day at 0800, and in those twenty-four hours, you might see sixty to ninety patients. Most cases were relatively simple problems, a middle ear infection or a sore throat. Others were acute—pharyngitis, urinary tract infections, and the like.

I had my initial three weeks of intensive Army indoctrination at Fort Sam Houston in San Antonio, Texas. On the second day, the members of our class—physicians, dentists, veterinarians, and other healthcare workers—were ushered into a large auditorium. The law at the time mandated that physicians be drafted for two years of obligatory service, which is how all of us came to be in that auditorium that day.

At the podium, a wiry, tough-looking sergeant-major appeared, and as he spoke into the microphone, his voice made it clear that he was in charge. His crisp, concise address seemed designed to motivate us to action or at least to the realization that we were now a cog in the wheel of the United States Army and not under civilian control. He kept his speech short:

> "Gentlemen, I am sure that it is your opinion sitting there that you will not be in a war during the time you are in the military. We understand that; however, you are wrong—totally incorrect. Let me straighten out your thinking. If you look at

the history of the United States, you will observe that we have been in a war about every twenty years or so. If you think that is going to change, you are wrong."

I looked at the man's uniform: He had service stripes all the way up one arm. However, the only way I could understand how he could have gotten them was to have enlisted at the age of sixteen. Needless to say, it was clear that he had been in the service for decades. He, of course, was correct about the frequency that our country finds itself at war too. He had my attention:

"I suggest, therefore, that for the next three weeks you listen intensely and try to remember what you learn as it may save your life."

The Sergeant-major then told us about the medical officers captured during the recent Korean War—and how, unable to read a map, many had fatefully gone in the wrong direction toward the enemy! He next directed us to complete two documents:

"You will complete these *now*! These will be signed and dated appropriately."

One of the documents was a power of attorney; the other, a will. There was no time for us to think about what they represented, though some were taken aback by his commanding tone. Many of the people in that audience—especially the doctors—weren't used to being talked to in such a manner, much less ordered about. Some looked startled, and others, insulted.

This was our introduction to the U.S. Army.

For me, this new reality came as no great surprise as I had always lived in a place where death was only one millimeter away. The same could not be said for my peers. For them, army culture was a shock, a great shock.

The majority of our group were psychiatrists who had lived cushy, protected lives on predominantly the East or West Coast with the normal and usual prejudices that some such people have against midwesterners and fly-over country. One might say they had never been exposed to the *real world of medicine*. After spending some time with them, I couldn't help wondering if they had ever been exposed to the *real world* at all—a good many of them appeared both unrealistic and narcissistic. At the least, they seemed used to being catered to and treated like royalty.

Having come out of the Great Depression and worked my way through college and medical school, I was not. From what I observed of them during indoctrination, this was as close to hell as they would normally have gotten in their lifetime: In the middle of Texas, in the furnace blast of summer, being told to fill out forms as if they were grade-schoolers. I suspect for many of them, the last two years had mostly been spent pushing papers. As I got to know them, this initial impression was only reinforced.

The noncommissioned officer who directed our activities told us to go into San Antonio and buy two sets of fatigues. The smart aleck boys from the coasts only bought one set so they could spend the leftover on something else. I did the exact opposite. I learned early on to do what I was told because the NCOs knew more about the upcoming days than I did. As for my two sets of fatigues, I ended up needing both when we found ourselves at Camp Bullis in the middle of nowhere, desolate even for rural Texas.

Thick, overgrown brush made it all but impossible to see more than several feet in any direction. Nonetheless, we were taught to read a map and use a compass—without which airplanes, ships, and spacecraft would not be able to accurately navigate along the four main compass directions of north, east, south, and west.

Then we were dropped off in pairs in the wilderness with several cans of rations and a canteen of water. We were given our coordinates on a piece of paper and expected to find our way back to the gathering area by nighttime for dinner. My partner and I had both listened carefully and followed the instructions given; we made it back for dinner with little difficulty. There was no one to help you if you hadn't listened or got lost! Those who got lost stayed out in the brush with the rattlesnakes and armadillos until morning, at which time someone came and picked them up. The exercise was made worse by a heavy rain storm, as only a Texas rain can fall. The deluge turned the ground into such a quagmire that we ended up having to push the trucks through the mud. By day's end, everyone who had made it back was cold soaked, caked with mud, and exhausted. The only relief was a field shower, which I used to contend with the mud. I can hardly describe the absolutely superb sensation of taking a field shower and crawling into my warm, dry, freshly laundered second set of fatigues before hitting my cot. I never figured out how my peers of the one set of fatigues—now wet and caked in mud—endured that night, especially on cots with only a piece of canvas under them. The moral of the story: Listen to the sergeant. Follow his instructions!

* * * * *

At Fort Sam Houston, we were introduced to *military medicine*, and the purpose of medicine took a subtle, but

definite change from attempting to deliver the best individual patient care possible. I found the reactions of my
fellow physicians during this transition to be fascinating.
Slowly but surely, we transitioned to this new medical per-
spective best depicted by the Army Medical Corps' slogan
at that time:

Preserve the fighting strength.

We all came to realize that, yes, we were doctors—however, we were no longer called to try to heal and decrease
the suffering of our fellow human beings. No, our aim
now was to preserve the strength of the military, of the
fighting force. This, of course, makes sense in the context in which we were operating: If your unit is taken, the
enemy is not going to provide you with the medical care
Americans have come to expect in their daily lives. Or
even in their military units. I could tell that some of my
contemporaries found this all rather repugnant.

Our training saw us running through a closed com-
bat course, firing thirty-caliber carbines from our left hips,
while advancing in line and in pairs at a slow walk—before
a noncom whose job was to be sure that we stayed in the
line. The point being, if you stayed in a line and fired to
the left, you weren't going to hit anybody.

It seemed simple. As I progressed down the field, I heard a noncom screaming obscenities, including some I had never heard before, at the doctor to my right. I could hear the thirty-caliber slugs zipping past my legs. Yet I couldn't stop; doing so would endanger the man to my left. We reached the other side intact, with a new appreciation for the way a terrified person with a weapon can become a menace to others.

On another night, our training escalated to dodging explosives on an infiltration course. Log bunkers had been filled with explosives and placed in a line, and our job was to crawl between the bunkers, despite some of the passageways being obstructed by logs. One could crawl around the ends of the logs, but this required a lot more effort than going over them. We were taught how to do the latter. This entailed straddling the log, tucking one's arms tight, and heaving oneself over. The idea was to land on the other side on your back with arms still tucked tight.

Following instructions, I found myself on the other side of the logs on my back, watching the tracers go by overhead—yes, this was a live ammunition exercise. I had been told there was always some eager beaver who, upon landing on the ground, jumped up too fast and got himself shot, and I vowed not to be that guy. Once I got over the logs and safely down in the ditch, I focused on the interesting things going on in the field before me. Apparently, I was the only one of us to opt for the straddle-the-log approach—everybody else appeared to have crawled around the logs. This was safer but not nearly as fun or as much of a challenge.

* * * * *

I had been assigned to Fort Campbell, Kentucky, with another physician from the East Coast who was an internist/gastroenterologist. Paul was of the Jewish faith and I was a Protestant; we became fast friends. When we arrived at Fort Campbell, our immediate commanding officer, Lieutenant Colonel Paulus, said, "Which of you two guys is gonna take them damned women off my back?" Unaware we had *damned women* in the U.S. Army, I was taken aback by the request.

The Colonel was an old Army man who had fought in World War II in North Africa and gone on to medical school under the aegis of Uncle Sam and the U.S. Army. He was male-soldier oriented. However, a large number of dependents were also attached to the base, and they were neither all males nor soldiers, but could still become ill and require hospitalization. At the time of our exchange, Paulus had two wards filled with female dependents that he had been taking care of, without any relief, while we were being trained, and he had had enough. I volunteered to take care of his *damned women* and proceeded to do so essentially by basically a civilian practice and ward within the military hospital.

I took on other duties too, such as being Officer of the Day. We started our day at the hospital at 0700 and left the next afternoon at 1700 or 1800 hours. That is correct—no time off, no sleep. We just worked and saw anywhere from seventy-five to a hundred patients come through the emergency room. Thank the good Lord for penicillin! There were multiple children who arrived with *otitis media* (ear infections), strep throat, and other routine ailments.

One of the more interesting cases was a corpsman who had been decorated in Korea several times. He was an excellent corpsman and a real example to the soldiers, particularly the other black soldiers. We became quite good friends, and one day I asked him if he thought there was any way I could get a particular type of desk for my office.

"What do you need, Doc?"

I described the desk I wanted and explained it didn't appear to be on the Army table of organization and equipment, which dictates what equipment can be used to staff a unit. The corpsman seemed to consider my question.

"Give me a couple of days, Doc, and I'll get it for you."

The Thinking Doctor

"How are you going to do that?" I asked.

He replied, "Oh, don't worry about it—and don't ask."

Several days later, the desk appeared in my office one morning completely installed. When I asked the corpsman how it had come to be acquired, he said, "You really don't want to know that information, Doctor."

That day, I learned a big lesson—trust your sergeants and other noncoms. This same corpsman had the misfortune of later ending up in the emergency room with nausea, vomiting, and diarrhea. He was given a shot of Compazine, or prochloroperazine, after which he suddenly began to develop peculiar posturing of his head, neck, and tongue. He appeared to have gone insane. The staff psychiatrist saw him and said that the corpsman was seriously ill from a psychiatric standpoint.

The psychiatrist—not being someone who liked to follow up on his patients after diagnosis—then proceeded to write his conclusion out in longhand. With copies made, he left the case for others to handle. This all happened over the course of one night, and I was unaware of it until the corpsman appeared on my ward as a patient the following morning. I no more than asked him what had happened, than it became clear to me that all of his symptoms had cleared, that he had no psychiatric abnormality and was, in fact, quite normal and ready to return to duty. He had had a not uncommon reaction to Compazine. This had produced his dystonic type of reactions, including the bizarre positioning of his body, the protruding tongue, and the unusual neck positions. This was good news.

The bad news was that the poor guy now had a report saying he was "psychotic, crazy" on his formal medical file.

The question now was: How would I handle this?

Fortunately, all the case copies were in my control. Suffice it to say that all of these copies quickly disappeared from his file as if the psychiatry consultation had never occurred. In the U.S. military if there is no record of it, it didn't happen. Hence, my corpsman went back to duty and everyone was happy.

I remained amazed at how making a thing or two disappear could improve a man's life—from being labeled a crazy, incompetent person who should be discharged from the military to being once again a competent leader of men at the snap of a finger (or loss of a form).

* * * * *

One Monday morning, in the same ward as the incident with the corpsman, I arrived only to be told of an incident that had happened over the weekend. Seems a hospitalized young sergeant had gotten out, bought a fifth of whiskey, and brought the bottle back to the ward where he had proceeded to get a new young private stone-cold drunk. The young private became critically ill, vomited repetitively that night, and remained badly hung over.

By the time I came in that morning, everyone had sobered up enough to be able to walk and eat, but was still feeling poorly. My head corpsman pointedly told me what had occurred. As a military officer, and thus the chief in charge, I was expected to discipline the sergeant for what he had done.

Monday went by, and then Tuesday. Both days I made rounds and remained cordial to the sergeant, but the tension on the ward was tangible as I went from one bed to the other checking on patients. At the end of my rounds, my corpsman approached me again.

"What are you going to do about the situation, Doc? You can't just let it go."

"Of course not," I replied. "I am thinking about it."

He looked at me incredulously. He was accustomed to military personnel making decisions immediately, which in his defense was usually the proper order of things.

The following day as I made rounds, I again said nothing to either of the two men. It was by then three days since the incident, and everyone on the ward had begun to believe that nothing of consequence was going to happen to anybody. However, the next morning as I made my rounds, I said to the perpetrator, "Sergeant, meet me in my office when I finish rounds."

"Yes, sir!"

I finished rounds, went to my office, and sat down at the desk. The sergeant appeared at the door, stepped inside, saluted, and remained at attention as if to emphasize the difference in rank. "Relax, sit down," I said.

He sat, completely disarmed and visibly surprised.

I ignored him and continued to busy myself with the papers I had been working on for another few minutes. Finally I pushed them aside, put my pen down, and looked at him straight on. Never taking my eyes off of him, I asked, "What happened the other day?"

He looked at me blankly and evidenced no knowledge of what I was talking about. Irritated, I looked harder at him and said, "Okay, stop lying. I know all about it. I have known about it for three days. You are not going to get away with anything. Do you want to be straight with me, or do you want to play games?"

He looked at me, startled, and quickly tried to justify himself and his behavior.

"Oh, stop it," I said. "There is no excuse for what you did—getting that poor, innocent boy drunk. You are supposed to be a leader of men, not a high school adolescent."

I then reviewed the events of the weekend as they applied to him and pointed out that he was a disgrace not only to the United States Army but also to himself. I said he ought to be ashamed because leadership was what being a noncom was all about, and he had failed as a leader.

The young man began to shuffle his feet, his eyes cast down to the floor. My line of approach appeared to be making an impression on him. I then asked him, "If you were sitting here with bars on your shoulders, and I was sitting where you are with stripes on my arm, what would you do to me?"

The look on his face made it clear such a thought had never crossed his mind nor had such values. His face paled and he looked frightened. I suspect no one in the chain of command had ever asked him to think about such a possibility before.

"I don't know, sir."

I knew he was lying. He knew exactly what he would have done in the same place: he would have taken my stripes away. I let him think about that for a moment.

Then I said: "You know, I can take those stripes away from you with one sentence. I can have you court-martialed."

He looked at me, and his eyes said that he thought that was what I was about to do.

Then I said, "I can do that. I can bust your rank, but I am not going to do that."

He now looked confused. I didn't blame him. He had expected immediate discipline—black and white, no gray. Instead, someone was sitting there talking to him about shame and responsibility and what it means to be a non-com. I suspect he had never been treated this way before. He appeared to hold his breath, seemingly unsure of what might happen next.

"I am not going to take your stripes, because I think the point here is to teach you a lesson—to make a man out of you."

He looked up at me stunned. *His stripes were safe?*

"However," I continued, "when you to go back on the ward, if you say one single word about what transpired in this office—and believe me, I know everything that happens here, I will bust you in rank. You can count on that. Do you understand?"

"Yes, sir!"

"You are *not* to leave the ward," I added. "No Red Cross girls, no library visits, nothing. You are just to sit on that ward. You can watch television." (The TV was an eight-inch black-n-white one.)

In the end, that is what happened. He went back to the ward, didn't say a word, and we went about our business.

The next morning, the mood on the ward was electrifying as I walked in. All anyone knew was that he had been called in to see me and afterward had refused to say a word to them about the meeting. To my surprise, the rest of the soldiers in the ward appeared frightened by how this had all played out—maybe because it was such a foreign outcome to them.

As for me, I could only hope that what I had done had made a man out of the young sergeant—and maybe a leader, as well. It has been my experience that in such situations, being right sometimes means reining in anger and trying to see the bigger, long-term picture.

* * * * *

Some of the most interesting cases I saw in the military came in via the venereal disease clinic. This was a different time. During duty on the artillery impact range, troops were bivouaced out to the boonies of Kentucky where the locals ran a whorehouse in a nearby town. On the weekends, the locals hauled a trailer out to the troops to serve as a portable brothel. Despite the casualness of this routine, it was forbidden by law and by command. Money, however, does talk. Sadly, this contributed to a rather high frequency of venereal disease for those who participated.

While known to everybody up and down the chain of command, this was yet another incidence of *something that happened but never happened*, so no discipline, repercussions, or reports to law enforcement were required. The unspoken agreement seemed to be that as long as it went on quietly and without any problems, nothing needed to be said. The assumption being that everyone was happy with the status quo. For better or for worse, this accommodation of brothels and bases, with the former in close proximity to the latter, is almost as old as war itself.

One story stands out from my time in the boonies. I will tell it just as it happened, so that it is factual rather than judgmental. Assigned to the Venereal Disease Clinic one Monday morning, I walked in to find a line of noncommissioned personnel lined up in uniform. At the sight of me, they snapped to attention; I immediately ordered them to be at ease. "What do we have here?" I asked my corpsman.

"They are all positive, Sir."

And he was right, each and every smear of the pus from their penises revealed the diplococci of gonorrhea.

At the time, the normal treatment for gonorrhea was a course of penicillin, with recovery ensuing promptly. (This is no longer true, as gonorrhea has now become resistant to nearly all antibiotics, save for one last recommended and effective class, cephalosporins.) I looked up and down the line of military personnel and said, "You all understand that you have gonorrhea?"

All but one big, tall, lanky private nodded.

I told the men to take the penicillin, drink plenty of water, and stay away from women for at least three days. As gave out the penicillin, I noticed the one private was still standing apart from the others. He looked at me and said, "Captain, *Suh*, do you means I got the *gomorrhea*?"

His deep accent made it clear that he was most likely from the deep South. "Yes, that's correct; you have gonorrhea. If you take your treatment, you will be fine."

There was a moment or two of silence; then, with an intense expression on his face, he said, "*Suh*, I can't have no gomorrhea!"

A little surprised, I asked, "Why not?"

"Don't you get the *gomorrhea* from them women?"

"Yes, that is the usual way."

"I ain't been near no women for six weeks, *Suh*."

I replied, "Well, that is not very likely. I am aware of what happens with those mobile units that come out to service you guys, so no need to pretend. Now, why don't you take your penicillin and get this over with so you can get back to duty."

My request did not appear to sit well with the private. Indeed, he became quite agitated. The other twenty-nine soldiers were done by now but still in line, waiting to be given permission to leave but unable to do so only because this one soldier kept insisting that he "a*in't got the gomorrhea.*"

Then suddenly a change.

I watched as the most wonderful smile slowly spread over the young man's face—to the point that his entire body seemed to be smiling. He looked at me knowingly and said, "*Suh,* I knows how I got the *gomorrhea.*"

"Great, tell me how you got the gonorrhea, and know that you do not get it from toilet seats."

My words did not deter him.

"Well, *Suh,* I was sittin' on the latrine out in the field, and you know how the latrine is; it has a raised mound of dirt with the potty on the top. I was usin' that. It was a hot day and I remembers it well. As I was sittin' there in the sunlight, thinking, I looks up and over the screen comes a big ol' fly. This big ol' fly comes over the screen and circles me over and over. Then it lands on my *peckuh,* and *dat's* the way I got the *gomorrhea.*"

The briefest moment of silence followed his declaration, and then I began to laugh so hard I was having trouble keeping my composure. My corpsman had been sitting nearby on a stool and overheard this exchange and burst out laughing with such vigor that he fell to the floor. The soldiers in line had heard the private's take as well, and they doubled over with convulsing laughter. If the young private had told this story as a comedy club contestant, he would have won the prize.

Finally, after everybody had quieted down to a normal state of decorum, instead of arguing, I said, "Okay, son, take your penicillin, and follow my instructions, and you will be just fine."

And, as far as I know, he was.

To this day, the gonorrhea outbreak incident remains my favorite story from my time in the military.

* * * * *

In the military, when antibiotics such as tetracycline came in, they came in by the thousands in tablet form. We used tetracycline for cases of nonspecific urethritis or occasionally gonorrhea when the patient couldn't take penicillin.

And then we didn't.

"Doctor, those pills you gave me went straight through me and were a nice, bright yellow in my bowel movements. I'm not absorbing them," one soldier said. He wasn't wrong. The pills that the military had bought were pressed so hard and coated so thoroughly that the tablets literally went through the patients intact. I am told that this is not supposed to happen. Our response was not immediate, but we did finally add to our instructions to carve an *X* on the tablets before taking them. Our cure rate rose by almost 100 percent overnight.

Sometimes it pays to listen.

* * * * *

My last case in the military involved my longest standing patient. She died in February of 2019, but when we met she was a young military wife in her twenties. Her husband was a sergeant-major of the 101st Airborne Unit, the top noncommissioned level in the U.S. Army. She came to see me because of headaches. She was not pleased with me at first; I was a new doctor and that irritated her, and probably rightly so. New military doctors, particularly with the low rank of captain, are not thought to possess much intelligence medically!

Maybe that was why she didn't wait for me to do any doctoring but rather immediately demanded that I refill the prescription of pills for her headaches.

My reply to her demand was that "I don't just fill prescriptions. I need to know something about you."

Her response was "Just give me my medicine and let me go. That's what everybody else does."

I replied, "Well, first of all, I am not everybody else, and secondly, I need to know something about you. Tell me how long you have had headaches."

She said she had been having the headaches for a long time and was taking methobamate for them. This drug is both a sedative and muscle relaxant, and I was reluctant to continue it without some good reason to do so. However, when I asked her for more information about her symptoms, she retorted that she would report me to the commanding officer of the base. "Feel free," I said. "The Army doesn't tell me how to practice medicine."

This seemed to give her pause.

I filled the conversational lull by saying, "Now, why don't you sit down and talk to me for a few minutes. I am sure we can come to some agreement. That medicine you're taking generally is not used for migraines."

As I looked closer, she appeared, despite her actual age, like an older woman with aged *facies*. She was pale and a little slow in some of her responses. Her skin was sallow. Likewise, her voice was not the usual high-pitched female voice of someone in her late twenties. She had had no pregnancies and little breast development.

"Tell me how often you have menstrual periods," I said.

Visibly furious, she screamed at me, "I don't have to tell you anything! I don't want to talk about that."

"Okay," I replied. "You don't tell me; I don't give you medicine. It's up to you."

She looked at me for a few minutes, reconsidered, and finally said, "Well, I had *menarche* (the start of menstrual periods) at a normal age. They stopped after several years, and I have not had any since."

"That's what I suspected," I said.

At this time in the history of medicine, we only had three diagnostic tools short of pneumoencephalograms or arteriograms, which were major endeavors. Those three tools were skull X-rays, EEGs, and lumbar punctures, or spinal taps. This was 1959, not present day.

Thyroid tests were primitive, but hers showed little thyroid activity (hypothyroidism). Her next tests were for adrenocortical function, and these levels were also reduced. It seemed clear to me that she had *panhypopituitarism*. In layman's terms, she had lost the pituitary function that makes the hormones that drive the thyroid, adrenal glands, ovaries, and more. All were absent or reduced.

Given her headaches, I suggested that the next step would be to get some X-rays of her skull. Sure enough, the *sella turcica*, the place where the pituitary gland lies, was extremely large. We then checked her vision carefully.

Eventually, we found the culprit, a tumor. We had caught the tumor early enough that it had not yet enlarged to the size that it altered her vision by encroachment upon her visual fields.

I sent her to a gynecologist who reported an infantile uterus and an atrophic vaginal wall. (Most women with estrogens have a thickened vaginal wall.) The gynecologist did a vaginal smear and found that she had no estrogen affect in the epithelium or the lining of the vagina. Her breasts also had little actual breast tissue. I explained all of this to her, and then referred her to my neurosurgical colleague from Vanderbilt University in Nashville, one Dr. Arnold Murowski. Being at a university teaching hospital, he was able to run many more tests.

A former chief neurosurgeon during the Korean War, Dr. Murowski had done fascinating studies on post-traumatic epilepsy. He was a delightful gentleman to work with. He saw my patient, looked at the film, and agreed with the diagnosis of a large pituitary tumor, one that had expanded enough as to destroy the normal pituitary function, as the studies indicated.

Our patient headed to Vanderbilt where the tumor was treated with radiation. We both monitored her visual fields, and were glad to observe no adverse changes associated with the reaction of the tumor to radiation. Even better, her headaches cleared. We then replaced her thyroid hormones, adrenocortical hormones, and estrogens.

Afterward, her husband came to me rather sheepishly and asked to talk with me in private. I, of course, said, "Great, tell me what the problem is, Sergeant-major."

"Well, as you know, we have not had children," he said. "She never gets pregnant, despite all of our efforts."

Very carefully (and as tenderly and kindly as I could), I told him that his wife did not have the hormonal apparatus to support a pregnancy to term.

I went on to explain that her uterus was infantile in size and probably would not change much without treatment, and even treatment might not work. Therefore, she would probably never become pregnant.

If this sounds incorrect medically now, remember that we were having this discussion in a medium-level military facility in 1959. My words at the time appeared to shock her husband, but he also seemed to accept my assessment. I suggested that they adopt children.

After my patient's husband was discharged from the service, they returned to Oklahoma, her birthplace. The tumor remained well controlled, and she never had a clinical recurrence or any complications thereof, with the exception that she was never able to have children. Many years later, after her husband had died, she returned to see me as a patient. I followed up with her until several years ago—a cantankerous beginning that ended with her being my longest standing patient. There's a lesson there for both physicians and patients, I think.

* * * * *

During my time in the military, I developed my own medical issue: pain in the right-lower quadrant of my abdomen with a general feeling of malaise and fatigue and an elevated white blood cell count. The physicians concurred on the probable diagnosis—*amoebiasis*, an intestinal illness caused by a parasite—but only after obtaining my medical history and learning I had spent some time in rural Mexico. I was put on quarters—basically confined to my room—while they poured medication into me. Unfortunately, I didn't respond to the treatment. Then before the date of my operation, I had a flare-up while the senior surgeon tapped to operate on me was out of town. The bird colonel who ran the hospital stepped in, opened me up, and found a ruptured appendix behind walled off the cecum. The operation was successful; the patient back to duty in one week.

I wish I could say that being a patient came with an epiphany with regard to patient care, but if there was one, I don't remember it.

* * * * *

The funniest opportunity that ever came to me while in the military, presented itself over a serving of fish.

The medical corps and medical service corps officers were seated at a large table with some of the nurses and dietitians. One dietitian, Major Nick, was seated across the table from me. I knew her well as we attended the same Bible study group on base.

As we finished lunch, I turned and addressed her, "Major Nick, thank you so much for singling me out for such recognition."

With that I had the ear of not only Major Nick but also the entire table, and all of them wore the same quizzical look on their face as I addressed her again. "I noticed that you made a particular point to have this piece of fish served to me, and I appreciate the honor."

Necks craned as the officers, nurses, and dietitians strained to see what gastronomical honor had been bestowed upon me. On my plate one dead cockroach could be seen in perfect relief against the cheese sauce. I had carefully eaten my fish around it so that the bug stood out in perfect silhouette.

Major Nick blushed scarlet; laughter ensued, and that was the end of that lunch!

* * * * *

Many a phone call has been known to change the course of a day. One afternoon, a call came in from one of the military gynecologists who quietly asked, "Do you know about anything weird that happens to women when they take vaginal suppositories?"

A bit bemused by his question, I replied, "No, I am not aware of anything."

I thought that might be that, but he persisted. "Well, this woman came in with *monilial* (yeast) *vaginitis*. I gave her the suppositories as they are usually tolerated well and work great."

"Yes, I am aware of that," I replied.

"Well, the young woman took the suppositories home, used them, and then came back and said she couldn't stand the suppositories. They were making her bleed and hurt like crazy, and she refused to use them anymore. Do you know of any neurological condition that would do this? There has got to be something to this," he said.

"No, I can't think of anything neurological that would do that," I said. "It sounds like it is related to the suppositories in some way."

Together, we went back and interviewed the patient again. She was a young, uneducated, married backwoods girl. Unable to read, she had used the suppositories as the doctor had instructed. Unfortunately, his instructions

179

had not included taking off the tinfoil cover on the suppositories. So she didn't, and she ended up with vaginal lacerations from trying to insert them.

In her defense, she tried to follow the doctor's orders—illiteracy just made it impossible to do so without error.

I suggested that perhaps opening the foil envelopes before putting the suppositories in would take care of the problem.

* * * * *

The suppository story reminds me of another unfortunate incident—only this one was not complicated by illiteracy per se but by dialect.

An associate came to me saying that he thought his patient was having seizures.

"Why do you think that?" I asked.

"Well, she keeps talking about falling off the roof."

"Oh!" I said.

He had my attention.

I followed him back to his patient. After talking with her for a few minutes and asking some questions, I learned she came from deep in the hills of Appalachia. I motioned for my associate to step outside so I could speak with him in private.

I then quietly told him, "What she is telling you is that she is having her period. Where she comes from in Appalachia, *falling off the roof* is another way of saying *menstrual period*—it has nothing to do with seizures or convulsions."

Another medical mystery, solved.

Chapter Twenty-Three

Epilepsy Case

THIS IS THE STORY of a young man who had intractable epilepsy. He had been brought to me for an opinion because of his seizures, which were of a tonic (stiffening)-clonic (twitching) variety. They were also idiopathic—that is, no one knew why they occurred, despite the best studies that were available at the time.

He had been placed on the standard treatment of phenobarbital and Dilantin. No blood levels were checked to see if he was in the therapeutic range for control of the seizures. Given the side effects—ataxia (an unstable gait), nystagmus (abnormal eye movements), and slurred speech—he had more than adequate medication. Since those medications were not working, I tried other medications, including mysolin and Tegretol or carbamazepine, which were both relatively new antiepileptic drugs. These were tried in various combinations with monotherapy. Yet no matter what we did, his seizures remained intractable.

The patient was quiet, ultra submissive, appeared depressed, and seemed unable to uphold a normal lifestyle or keep a job. As he got older, he attempted various types of work and was routinely fired from them because of his seizures. Still, he persisted in trying to get and keep a job. By law he could not drive a motor vehicle, so this put a great deal of pressure on his parents.

Then one day I came upon literature regarding vagus nerve stimulators and their use for intractable epilepsy. The paradigm was that if one had tried various anti-epileptic drugs in several combinations that weren't effectively handling the situation further manipulation of drugs was of little or no use. (Sadly, this paradigm has not changed appreciably since that time.) The company producing the vagus nerve stimulator device was located near Houston. They invited me to come for training; I went down and learned how the device operated.

The transmitter was placed under the skin over the chest wall on the left side. A wire was run under the skin and up to the vagus nerve in the neck. A pre-stretched clip, encircling the vagus nerve was then placed. The device was controlled and programmed transcutaneously with a computer. No direct brain surgery was performed. Hence, not only was this treatment accepted by patients more readily, but there was also less morbidity and mortality associated with this treatment.

Using a hand wand, a doctor could program the length and intensity of the electrical discharge of the device as well as the frequency through the skin. Upon my return to Oklahoma City, I explained all this to the patient and his family; they were more than eager to go ahead. As nearly as I can determine, this man would be the first private neurology patient who had a vagus nerve stimulator implanted in Oklahoma City.

Only one thing remained to do. I needed to find a surgeon to implant the device. The procedure had never been done at any of the hospitals in Oklahoma City; the concept was *that* new. Fortunately, I found a young ear, nose, and throat surgeon who was more than eager to try.

He studied the procedure, and then went ahead and did the implant. The change in our patient's behavior was remarkable. He started to become much more outgoing and inquisitive. As the drug doses were reduced, he was able to walk without staggering or losing his balance—his speech no longer slurred and his cognitive ability improved. He now laughed and outwardly appeared to enjoy life rather than being muted and unresponsive. He and his family agreed the difference was like the difference between night and day.

Subsequently, he did have a few seizures, but these seemed to correlate to missed medication or meals that left him mildly hypoglycemic. As the years have passed, his seizure control has improved distinctly. He now drives a motor vehicle and is steadily employed.

At one point after the change, he told me that he was going to quit his job. This may sound like a small issue, maybe even a backslide moment to most readers, but it was in fact a major accomplishment for this young man. Before the implant, he had been fired from multiple jobs because of the seizures, and now he was going to quit his current one. He had become so confident of his seizure control that he was willing to take the risk of leaving one job to take another one.

The lesson to be learned is that a physician should never give up on a patient because he or she has not responded to the standard therapy. Physicians have a tendency to get locked into a pattern of conditioned response to diseases rather than pursuing individualizing treatment, which was done in the case of this young man.

Too often, they continue to use the standard treatments, which expose them to much less risk and certainly not to the criticism that can come for daring to try new and unusual plans of care. Some people in the community believed the VNS concept was a whole lot of quackery and that I was exercising poor judgment in suggesting the young man even try it.

Many of those same doctors remain unwilling to have their patients receive this treatment. They are locked into using the same regimen of drugs rather than considering the newer modalities, including deep brain stimulation, selective ablation of brain areas, and other emerging treatments.

Myself, I would rather remain a doctor who is also a continuing learner.

Chapter Twenty-Four

Experiences in Psychiatry

D URING THE YEAR of my Senior Neurology residency, I was also in charge of the closed—that is, locked—psychiatric ward. One is not put in a locked ward unless his or her behavior is so disorganized or dangerous that the locks on the doors are necessary. I found some patients actually looked forward to being moved into such a ward, seeing it as a safe harbor from the outside world. Most patients, however, resented the loss of their personal freedom to move around as they pleased.

What I found interesting was that I had no problem relating to these patients. I could walk into a room with the most violent patient, sit down, and start to talk, and the patient would relax, sit down with me, and engage in conversation. To be very clear, this conversation may have comprised only of a recounting of their delusional and hallucinatory experiences, but at least was done without severe emotional outbursts or threatening motor behavior.

There were, of course, exceptions.

On one such occasion, I took a right jab to the jaw that sent me across the room and to the floor. As I explained to the shocked junior resident helping pick me off the floor, "That's the way it is. This is life here."

But such violence was the exception, and I found the routine days filled with sitting and listening to the patients to be fascinating. I still remember the stories of one locked unit patient, a prominent wealthy male patient who hailed from Chicago.

With such patients, the need to help them carefully sort out reality from unreality in their delusions is critical. The physician simply serves as a facilitator to the patient to do this—to present the workings of his or her psyches. To hear this successful college-educated man talking about how the government had wired his home's electrical outlets so it could listen in on his conversations or send messages over his television to brainwash him was *riveting*. Such accounts were always presented in an earnest manner.

They were the patient's reality. He was 100 percent convinced that his hallucinations and delusions were real, and they were elaborate ones!

According to this gentleman (and many others I treated in the unit), the FBI had assigned multiple special agents to watch every movement of his car, his chauffeur, or his maid. They all believed that the FBI listened to his conversations on a regular basis via electronic wall plugs. They always had a reason as to why the special wires on the television set, on the radio, on the electrical outlets, lamps, or telephones couldn't be seen or found—often claiming that the devices were so small and cleverly hidden that they couldn't be detected with the human eye. Some even thought the hospital food was poisoned with truth pills.

At the time, the only treatment available for such patients was electric shock or insulin coma. Both of these were accompanied by a certain element of risk. One must try to imagine what a paranoid, delusional individual must think when he or she is restrained or shocked with electricity to the brain. Sadly, the reasoning for said treatment cannot always be understood by the patient, given that the context of the treatment is clearly verifying and proving the patient's paranoia. The locks on the doors proved likewise.

I recall one young resident who became convinced that his patient was telling the truth—that the physician and police were, in fact, in cahoots against him. With a certain amount of time and difficulty, I was able to convince him that if one looked at the totality of what the patient related as his reality, it became clear that his perception was delusional and did not fit into a normal paradigm.

There was, however, one interesting related case of a postal employee. This patient thought he was being spied on at work. The fact of the matter was that he *was* being watched very closely. Apparently, as we understood it, he worked at the branch of the local post office that handled highly classified mail and parcels with valuable contents. There was, in fact, an observation point in the building from which people who handled these sensitive materials could be monitored. To do otherwise would have abdicated the responsibility of the U.S. Postal Service.

There was some truth in his perception, if one listened to this patient, though it quickly became clear that he was paranoid delusional in regard to his work situation, which was reasonable—but also to outside situations, which was not reasonable and could not be verified. As the reader can understand, discretion had to be observed in all of these matters, and patient statements—no matter how outlandish—needed to be investigated carefully for verification or lack thereof.

Much of this would change with the advent of new psychotropic drugs. The first one being Thorazine, or chlorpromazine.

Thorazine is a potent drug that delivered a verifiable breakthrough for patients in decreasing psychotic behavior and delusional thinking. Since its arrival, there have been a number of much better products emerge with fewer significant side effects. These have changed the face of psychiatry. Now only rarely is electric shock given, and as for the insulin coma? It is gone.

Chapter Twenty-Five

Further Experiences in Psychiatry

ONE OF THE MOST interesting things about being a resident in the locked psychiatric ward for a year was that I saw patients return—often more than once. In the process, over time many of them became something more than patients. Maybe this was because being a psychiatric ward, one of our structural dynamics was providing a way that allowed the development of our patients' human relationships.

They might have been in a locked unit, but our patients still had hobbies that they were allowed to continue and explore, like handwork. I still have a set of hot pads made from intricate interlocked wooden components that I received. I was touched that a patient had thought enough of me to make and give me such a gift.

I believe my last anecdote in psychiatry is an unique one as I am not aware of another physician who has had such an experience. The patient was a middle-aged female who presented with severe psychosis, agitation, and a high fever, more than 104 degrees F.

My chief at the time immediately announced that we would "give her electric shock and get her well."

I remember looking at him with amazement before saying, "If you give her electric shock, you will probably kill her."

My reasoning presumed that the patient might have had a severe systemic infection first, and only then developed the psychosis. I wasn't alone in this belief; my fellow residents concurred, and thus were also diametrically opposed to the senior/controlling neurologist's call for electric shock therapy for the patient.

"How much time do you want to study her before we give her shock? We have to do it quite promptly."

I was still thinking *If you shock her, it will kill her*, but I replied, "Okay, give us twenty-four hours."

In that twenty-four hours, several of us examined the patient from one end to the other, including examination of all orifices, multiple blood tests, X-rays, and a review of her files. At the end of the twenty-four hours, her fever was still more than 103 degrees F., and she was obviously psychotic and becoming dehydrated, despite our ongoing efforts. At this point, the chief said, "Okay, we will shock her this morning."

To say that all of the house staff were fearful was to grossly understate the case. We began planning how to revive the patient after what we anticipated to be the lethal effect of the electric shock treatment—as well as how to tell her family that her demise had come from EST.

As ordered by the chief, the electric shock was administered, and an amazing thing happened. The patient's temperature dropped to 98.6 degrees F., basically normal! She also became cooperative and started to eat and drink.

The chief looked at us and said, "That's what I told you would happen, gentlemen." Then he added, "By this afternoon, her fever will be up, and we will have to give electric shock again in the morning."

That was exactly what happened, and by the next afternoon the patient's fever was 101 degrees F. She would go on to receive several more EST treatments. After that, she had no more fever, and her psychosis cleared, as did the agitation.

The lesson here is that doctors who have been doctors for a long time have seen a lot, and the chief had seen many such patients previously and knew exactly the type of schizophrenia represented in the woman and what its response to electric shock would be. If any psychiatrist in the 21st century used this technique, it would be considered either barbaric or at the least incorrect, suggesting even malpractice. However, once more, please remember that this was the 1950s. We did not have access to the potent drugs and procedures that exist now.

Still, treating this patient taught me a lesson, an important one at that. I learned that there existed medical professionals who knew a great deal more than I did—physicians who had better clinical, or psychiatric, judgment based on their experiences.

I tried to remember that going forward.

Chapter Twenty-Six

Mistakes

UNFORTUNATELY, in addition to missed diagnoses that occur in good faith, there are occasional cases of incorrect procedure and thinking that lead to bad diagnoses and bad outcomes for the patients. There were four in particular that left an impression on me.

The first involved a forty-year-old female executive whom I had treated for recurrent episodes of multiple sclerosis since she was in her twenties. She had first come in for a routine appointment, during which she confided, "Doctor, I have so much pain."

Generally, mild multiple sclerosis is not associated with severe pain. My first question was, "Where is the pain?" She pointed to the left lower quadrant of her abdomen and the *inguinal*, or groin, area on that side.

I asked, "Did you injure yourself or traumatize the area in any way?"

Her answer was no to both; the pain had developed over a period of time. After a careful examination, I found no evidence of a change in her neurological condition and told her, "I don't think this is neurological, but I will send you to a doctor who thinks."

She gave me a perplexing look and said, "Don't all doctors think?"

I answered, "Oh, of course not. Few physicians methodically think diagnostically of the possibilities before they launch into a plan of treatment."

As with most humans, and as I have said before, doctors tend to follow routines when a little curiosity would often serve them better. I sent her off to see a general surgeon, who was a good friend of mine and an excellent diagnostician.

He immediately realized because of her *ataxia* (imbalance) from the MS, she had developed an irregular, unstable walking pattern despite using a cane. This had produced a severe muscle sprain and, hence, the pain. He injected the groin area several times with steroids and a local anesthetic. She traded her cane for a walker to decrease the ataxia and improve her stability with walking.

This cured her painful problem.

* * * * *

The second case was somewhat more dramatic and worrisome. The patient was one I had seen for many years for a stable neurological condition until the day that she arrived at her annual checkup looking concerned.

"You know, Doctor, I have so much pain, and no one can figure out what is wrong with me."

"Where is this pain?" I asked.

She indicated that it was in the *suprapubic* area, the area above the pelvis in her lower abdomen. I asked what diagnostic procedures had already been attempted. There had been a couple. She had first gone to a gynecologist, who had done a PAP smear that came back fine and showing no sign of cancer. She had then gone to a gastroenterologist, who did a series of diagnostic studies, including a colonoscopy, only to tell her she was healthy. Neither the gynecologist nor the gastroenterologist had any explanation for her pain, which was her chief complaint. Neither had proposed any other diagnostic testing to find the source of it.

I had her lie down on the examining table, saying somewhat apologetically, "I don't do internal medicine any longer, but I think I need to examine your abdomen."

Sure enough, she had a mass about the size of a softball; it was easily palpable, above the *symphysis pubis*, or front of the pelvic bone. You didn't have to be much of a physician to feel something that large. I asked her, "Didn't anyone have you lie down and examine your abdomen since that is where your pain is?"

She looked at me, shook her head, and said, "No one ever examined my abdomen before you. They only did procedures or tests."

One put a speculum in her vagina and did a smear for cancer. The gastroenterologist did his scoping, as expected. Unfortunately, my observation would be that this type of medical mistreatment—the failure to do a thorough examination or even a *basic* examination of a patient—is becoming more common. We have become increasingly specialized, and in doing so have forgotten that the general practice of medicine involves the *whole patient*, not *only* the part that is being studied.

This case, sadly, came out badly. The woman had an ovarian carcinoma that killed her within a fairly short time. To paraphrase a quote by Sir William Osler, a great diagnostician of years past:

Listen to the patients; they will tell you the diagnosis.

My point is that this patient had *abdominal pain* that was new, and it needed to be examined and explained—not explained away by negative examinations. Listen to the patient! Do not stop without a reasonable diagnosis that can explain the presenting complaint.

* * * * *

The third case that I would like to share is that of a white, unmarried female about thirty-eight-years old. I saw her in my office for what she described as her *disfigured face*. Specifically, she stated that her nose looked terrible, and it seemed that no one could figure out what was wrong with it. She had been referred to me by another physician unable to ascertain the root of her perceived problem. The patient had already had three invasive procedures on her nose and the middle part of her face. At this point, her face still had acceptable contours; she would certainly pass for a female of her age. Nonetheless, her complaints were vociferous, repeated, and fit into a relatively stereotyped, repetitive pattern. She insisted, to put it mildly, that she had a "disfigured, horrible, disgusting" face. Her words, not mine.

Her description was predicated upon her concept of what her nose looked like, rather than any other feature. Her demeanor during her examination was that of a woman in great distress—someone filled with emotional tension, anger, and frustration. I did a neurological exam and also ordered imaging to be sure that we were not overlooking anything that was structurally significant. The tests were all negative, as was her neurological examination. I had to tell her that I could find no explanation for why her perception of her nose and face was so poor.

She reminded me that three surgeons had operated on her quite willingly because of the configuration of her nose. In her opinion, that meant that they must have seen something wrong with it or they would not have operated on her! In other words, the very fact that they had agreed to operate made her complaints *realistic* to her.

This stood in reverse to what one might consider reasonable. After her second visit and the imaging results, I began to grasp that we were dealing with someone who had a *somatic* delusion. I told her that in my opinion, no reason existed for further surgery, and she might consider living with her nose and face as they were. This did not deter her. She immediately said she would find someone else who would "fix her face and make it look good again." Given her anguish over a nose that she perceived as disfigured, reasoning with her was not possible. She was not listening to me on a reasonable, cognitive level.

Finally, I gave up and said, "I will send my reports to your referring doctor. Thank you, and have a good day." I then called the ENT surgeon who had sent her to me and told him why he should most certainly *not* operate on her again. My diagnosis was that she had Somatic Delusion Syndrome. The surgeon made somewhat noises about the need for surgery, saying she was disfigured. Furthermore, he firmly believed that he could give her relief! This is not an uncommon reaction from surgeons in my experience; their activities are predicated on the idea that they can improve, and not just stabilize, the situation by the use of the cut, tie, suture techniques of surgery.

As expected, the woman was operated on for the fourth time. A little while afterward, she returned to my office. This encounter was a repeat of the first, except that now all of her rage (that is what is was, *total rage*) fell on the, in her words, stupid, nasty, irresponsible surgeon who had dared to operate on her again only to fail to repair any of the damage. In her words, he had only made it worse. This reaction was to be expected, given that the perceived damage was psychological in origin and was in fact a profound, somatic delusion, or dysmorphism.

* * * * *

I was only indirectly involved with the fourth case in which the diagnosis was made incorrectly, but this case teaches yet another valuable lesson.

A young man had been studying the Bible—most specifically the old law given to Moses on the mount by God—that exhorts, "If your eye offends you, pluck it out." The patient took this to mean that if he looked at pornography, which he believed was evil, sinful, and deserving of the wrath of God, his *eyes* were at fault.

And so, he gouged out his own eye!

I cannot begin to conceive of how painful this must have been for him, but it sent him to the emergency room. An ophthalmologist saw him and repaired the damaged orbit as best he could. The young man left the E.R. with one working eye and unresolved psychiatric issues. If you thought the pain and ramifications of losing his eye had stopped his obsessive religious acts, you would be sorely mistaken. Instead, after some time went by, he appeared again in the emergency room, bleeding badly.

He had amputated his penis with a knife.

The self-induced penectomy had caused so much bleeding that he had been rushed to the emergency room so his wounds could be closed.

The point of this last story is that the ophthalmologist should have recognized the general medical and psychiatric nature of the young man's situation. Rather than simply addressing his particular specialty—that is, stabilizing the orbital morphology—he should also have insisted that the patient be hospitalized where he could be seen by a psychiatrist and possibly a priest, minister, rabbi, or other appropriate religious figure, given the reason behind his first attack on his body.

The ophthalmologist *did not* do this. Hence, we now had a young man with one eye and an amputated penis. I never heard what trauma the young man went on to endure after this self-harm, but it was clear to me that this should have been a case of single-minded malpractice, a failure to treat the whole patient.

We are called to be *thinking doctors*—to act as a physician, not a technician would act. The cost of not doing so is unnecessary tragedies such as these.

Chapter Twenty-Seven

Conclusion

S O, AFTER SPENDING sixty-one years in medical practice, primarily in neurology, the end has come. Retirement occurred for me in June of 2016. At the time of this dictation, I am still practicing one-half day a week in a free clinic, still with an emphasis on neurology. I continue to find it rewarding to provide assistance to patients who have few financial resources.

At age ninety-three, I believe that perhaps I can predict the future of neurology given the multiple decades I have spent in practice. Neurology has moved from what was once a descriptive practice of describing and classifying pathology to a therapeutic-driven specialty. This is welcomed, particularly in cases of multiple sclerosis, recurrent strokes, atrial fibrillation with embolization, and the like.

Sadly, the process of bringing such advancements to bear on a patient remains less than ideal. I still see too many patients who, when I ask them what their previous doctor said or did, tell me something akin to what happened in the four cautionary tales in the previous chapter:

Did the doctor take a thorough medical history?
No.

Did the doctor take the time to talk to you about where the pain was located, or when the pain appeared, or what has happened in your life recently that might have acted as a precursor to the ailment?
No.

Refusing to take the time to do such basic patient care, I believe, decreases the ability of the physician to think deeply and well about the case that has presented itself in the patient before the doctor—and thus the likelihood that the doctor will find a way to the proper diagnosis and treatment.

This keeps a physician from being a *thinking doctor*.

Yes, you can see more patients per hour per day, and yes, this increases the income of your medical group or hospital as well as your own personal income—but such an approach certainly does not make for the best outcomes for your patients. And, in my personal opinion, it is not the way to practice medicine. People are individuals, with unique medical backgrounds, and as such, they need to be treated as individuals, especially during what are often among the most critical moments of their and their loved ones' lives.

Your patients come expecting their doctor to use all the education, knowledge, and experience said doctor has collected to shine a light on their case.

One reason that I have always made it a habit to address each of my patients by his or her proper name, such as Mr. Jones, or Mrs. Smith, or Miss Brown, is because people expect a doctor to be professional and for the relationship to be mutually respectful.

Patients prefer that their physicians be professional and relate to them seriously as patients rather than good ole buddies. In my opinion, this calls for the physician to look like a physician. In other words, a doctor should be dressed properly for the environment, whether that includes a coat and tie or a white coat. A physician should look clean and neat may sound like your elementary school teacher or mother talking; nonetheless, I have found that patients find such things reassuring—maybe because they suggest an orderly disciplined approach to life and thus medicine.

Doctors should also learn to ask the patients questions that go beyond specific medical ones. They should ask older patients if they are retired, and if so, what they did for work. Most patients will be delighted to tell them, and the doctors will learn a lot on a personal level about not only the patient's mind but also possible health problems that might stem from the work the patient once did.

If a patient brings a relative or spouse in, the doctor should look at their relatives and speak to them as well — this recognizes the family members as important players in the process, which they are or may well one day be.

These days, one is often cautioned by management not to spend too much time with a patient! Yet despite being plugged into electronic medical records, physicians are not being rewarded for this with more one-on-one time with patients but are rather penalized or forced to act as a typist. I find one is rewarded not for the patients helped or the positive outcomes reached but rather reimbursed only for the number of patients seen, as if practicing medicine were like working on an assembly line. This is perverse and ultimately, in my opinion, has led to a clear deterioration in medical care in this country.

I believe it also contributes to physician burnout. Too many medical decisions are made by insurance companies or governmental agencies. These third parties too often have little or no interest in good medical care, continuing medical education, or physician-patient relationships. They are interested only in the bottom line; they are interested only in money and profits.

Sadly, the patients themselves have little way of knowing how adequate or inadequate the medical care that they receive is. They may be influenced to think that doing a series of tests gives them the proper diagnosis, but it often does not, as evident by the examples I provided earlier in this book.

Lastly, I think that, as a group, physicians have become less humanized. This is not meant as a derogatory or insulting statement to any physician. I have the greatest respect for my fellow physicians who are motivated by a desire to help people. I believe, however, that they have been handicapped in this process by the electronic record system and the fact that third parties are controlling patient access to not only physicians and medical care but also to medications as well.

Mine has been a wonderful lifetime of medicine. I remember to this day many patients and their stories in detail, and I hope that the reader will have enjoyed some of these stories and memories from a bygone era.

About the Author

Ernest G. Warner served in the U.S. Army
Medical Corps before spending sixty-five
years in a neurological practice. He makes
his home in central Oklahoma.